# I'LL NEVER BE HU

# SLIM
# SATISFIED
## AND SEXY AT 56

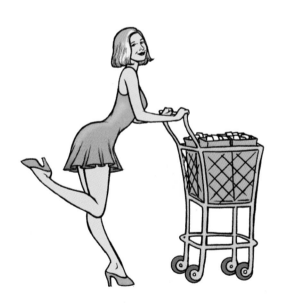

## BY F. CECIL & BOO GRACE

**Note:** With our weight control program, as with all weight control programs, it is advisable to consult with your physician.

PLEASE JOIN OUR E-MAIL LIST AT:
www.slimsatisfiedandsexy.com

FIRST EDITION

Copyright © 2008 F. Cecil Grace Publications

ISBN-10: 0-615-22892-5 · ISBN-13: 978-0-615-22892-1

To order additional copies, please visit Amazon.com

*Cover and interior design: Jeffry Braun*
*Interior illustrations: Russell Braun & Jeffry Braun*

Manufactured in the United States of America

# A Word from the Doctor

Boo's medical guru from the beginning has been Dr. Jonathan Epstein, MD. Many other doctors have added their support. Dr. Epstein writes: E-Mail, May 28, 2005

Satiation and weight loss? What once seemed impossible is now being espoused by reputable scientists as well as the mainstream media. You can eat more and lose weight at the same time. The science is sound, and the science is very simple. Boo has known this intuitively for a very long time. Eat plenty of delicious, filling, low-calorie healthy foods, as Boo has outlined, and you will lose weight. Moreover, she has created the tools to make your diet successful, and more important, she shows you how to *maintain* that weight loss for a lifetime. Boo's diet program is simple and healthy, yet sophisticated and revolutionary. Boo's diet program works. What's more, you will be happier because Boo has put an end to the hunger that plagues all other diets. I have had the pleasure of using (and thoroughly enjoying) Boo's products. I lost weight with Boo's program, and the weight has stayed off. I strongly encourage you to do the same.

Jonathan Epstein, MD

BS - Cell and Developmental Biology, University of Rochester
MS - Anatomy and Neurobiology, Boston University School of Medicine, 1995
MD - Boston University School of Medicine, 1999
Internship - Brown Rhode Island Hospital,
    affiliated with Brown University School of Medicine
Residency - Emergency Medicine, Long Island Jewish Hospital,
    affiliated with Albert Einstein University School of Medicine, 1999-2003
Board Certified in Emergency Medicine, 2004
Assistant Professor Emergency Medicine, Mount Sinai School of Medicine, 2006

# The Cure for Obesity At Last

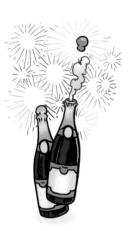

I HAVE THE CURE FOR OBESITY. I base my cure on foods that didn't exist a decade or two ago. Some dieters use Wonder Light bread, which is half the calories of ordinary Wonder Bread. It has the same taste and even more fiber. Others use 45-calorie Promise margarine instead of the 100-calorie product. No one to my knowledge, however, has created a comprehensive program of eating the new low calorie foods, which are delicious and filling.

We begin by asking what you desire to be your ideal weight. We multiply that number by thirteen for the normally active person. It takes about thirteen calories per pound of weight to maintain the bodily functions of breathing etc. If your ideal set point is 140 pounds we multiply 140 x 13 to get 1,820. As you make this your standard daily level of caloric intake your body will gradually make this your normal weight.

There are hearty souls among you who would like to jump start the process of getting to your ideal weight. For those heroic creatures we multiply by 10 instead of 13. The adventuresome person who wants to reach and maintain the 140 pound level quickly will make due on 10 calories per pound of weight ideal, 1,400 calories a day. On reaching the goal he or she would then slowly increase to the 13 calorie per pound level.

A woman weighing 160 pounds might aspire to drop 30 pounds. To do so quickly, she could eat only 10 calories per pound per day, based on the 130 pounds she plans to reach. During the transition period I put her on a program of 10 calories times her 130-pound ideal weight — or 1,300 calories a day. By using my recommended foods, she can be reasonably full even on 10 calories per pound of her goal weight during the transition period. Then, once she has reached her ideal weight, she can be really full, using my recommended foods, on the 13 calories per pound of her weight, which is my standard for maintenance.

These are our standard approaches. We aim for 10 calories per pound of ideal weight for the jump start dieter and 13 calories a pound for the standard dieter. There is still a third category of dieter. There is a group that is frightened of the new foods themselves and who are gun-shy of getting on any serious regimen of weight control. These are people who come from families with rigid food taboos. It would be wrong to minimize the power, even on the most intelligent person, of these rigid dietary fears. A Hindu may be an atomic scientist but he might be revulsed at the thought of eating beef. Many major Asian cultures eat dog meat. We Americans would rather starve first. On the other hand American mothers attacked canned foods when they were first produced. More recently my own grandmother viewed the new frozen foods with hostility. She was sure that new fangled foods were "full of chemicals" and "artificial." To the obese person of this background we would hold back on talking of 10 calorie or even 13 calorie programs. We introduce the new foods slowly over a period of weeks and months.

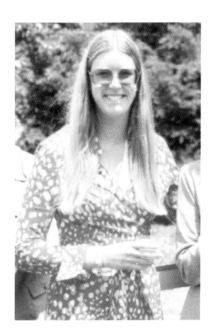

*My before picture*

This gradual transition gives the dieter immediate gratification. It also enlists the obese persons' desire for slenderness. There is much written about the terrible difficulty of losing weight. Dieting has been compared to kicking cigarette and drug habits. On the other hand by harnessing the ego's desire for slenderness we can overcome even the strongest family conditioning. We can take the most stubborn dieter by the hand and help him to take the leap of eating Wonder Light bread instead of the regular Wonder Bread.

Making this bread substitution means that you will get immediate gratification by realizing that you are losing between 120 and 200 calories a day. You may be frightened of this newfangled food. Your fear may be comforted by the knowledge that you are losing between a pound and a pound and a half a month by switching from Wonder to Wonder Light. The second week, or whenever you feel up to it, take another baby step: switch from butter or margarine to Promise Light or Promise Ultra. As a parallel step, change from frying with Wesson Oil or other vegetable oil to frying with Pam or similar spray. These two baby steps are even more potent in calorie reduction than the light bread. The third week, or whenever you might be ready, we ask you to substitute Kraft 10-calorie-per-tablespoon mayonnaise for Kraft 100-calorie-per-tablespoon mayonnaise. Not only would you cut calories by 90 percent, but you can be lavish in using mayonnaise on salads, such as tuna fish, egg, macaroni, potato, and coleslaw. The fourth week, heed the good mother and substitute your regular 60-calorie-per-tablespoon dressing with any of the standard low-calorie or calorie-free dressings. The fifth week, take the plunge of substituting fat-free cheese for regular cheese. By now, your taste is so refined that fat is beginning to be repulsive. You will revel in the taste of cheese that is full of flavor without the fat. Fat can actually clog the taste buds.

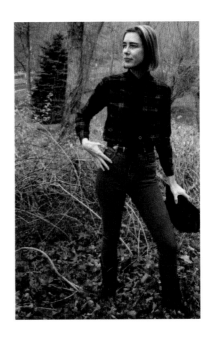

*My after picture*

At this point, you are ready to debunk the old sweetener myth. A Puritan family tradition has warned that saccharine, sucralose and aspartame cause cancer in laboratory animals. This old wives' tale has been disproved over and again. All the old warning labels about them have now been discarded. At their worst, it would have taken mountains of the artificial sweetener to cause any danger to laboratory animals. Humans would have had to drink oceans of soda sweetened with these products, and even then, there would have been no danger. The National Cancer Institute has said officially that presently available artificial sweeteners, including saccharine, sucralose and aspartame, hold no threat of cancer to anybody.

While the old wives' tale held sway, millions of kids and adults were getting fat drinking liquids like Classic Coke with about 10 teaspoons of sugar for a small cup. This old wives' tale about artificial sweeteners has caused children and adults to drink these sugar drinks and gain millions of pounds of fat. The cost in lives and amputations and sheer human misery is beyond my comprehension. How any mother or father can live in a home serving heaps of sugar to their innocent obese children is beyond my comprehension. I actually broke relations with a longtime friend when she insisted on serving regular Snapple to her obese children.

Superstition dies hard. You may find it a plunge to drink sodas made with artificial sweeteners. The savings in calories, however, will be astounding. Superstition can be a powerful force. Truth can be an even more powerful force. Those who scream danger at the old time fears of artificial sweeteners are urging parents and children to court the very real threat of diabetes. They are urging their families to become part of the 92 percent of the avoidable cases of diabetes and to become frontline candidates for lower limb amputations. Diabetes is the cause of a lower limb amputation every 30 seconds.

In succeeding weeks we will hold your hand as you switch to no- or low-calorie gravy, jelly and jam, syrup, milk, cream, and sour cream. As you adjust to the clean world of fat-free dining, we will hold your hand as you make quiche with Egg Beaters and cheesecake and pudding with minimal calories.

I cannot predict the specific amount of weight loss as I can predict it in our 10- and 13-calorie-per-pound programs. I can, however, assure you that your weight will plummet. Now that Atkins is passe, no reputable authority claims that there is any basis for weight control except calories. Eat more calories than you burn, and you will gain weight. Eat fewer calories than you burn, and you will lose weight. I have estimated that 12 small changes should result in a loss of at least 15,000 calories a month. This would come to about four pounds a month, my ideal rate of weight loss. The only deprivation to you is the loss of fat, which clogs the taste buds and the arteries and results in obesity.

# CHAPTER 1

# Slimming Down to Your Ideal Weight

## Calorie Outline and Sample Day
### 1,280 calorie outline — For the average American woman

Refer to Boo's menu choices to learn how to design your meals. The average American woman is 5 foot 3 inches tall. She should weigh 128 pounds. She consumes 13 calories per pound per day (1,664 calories). During the slimming-down period I keep her full on 1,280 calories per day (128 x 10 =1,280). She will remain full while losing about a pound per week — the ideal pattern of weight loss. The calories at each meal are approximate, but the day's total should not exceed 1,280 during the slimming-down period.

The decrease of calories during the slimming-down period could be achieved gradually. I have found, however, that your enthusiasm in beginning my Fullness Program and the knowledge that this is an exciting new lifestyle give your psyche such a lift that your body does not hang on to the old weight as you drop calories.

Once you have slimmed down, it is desirable to return to the normal 13 calories per pound of your ideal weight in a gradual manner. Once you have reached your ideal weight, start adding 50 calories a day until you are at 1,664 calories. If, on a given day, your weight shoots up, either stay at the same calorie level or drop back 50 calories. Be patient and confident, and your weight will stabilize at its ideal point. You may even, like me, have difficulty keeping your weight up to your ideal level.

## Calorie Outline and Sample Day

**1,280 calorie outline — For the average American woman (continued)**

| | |
|---|---|
| Breakfast | 160 cal |
| Midmorning snack | 100 cal |
| Lunch | 140 cal |
| Gold coins | 120 cal |
| Tea Sandwich | 100 cal |
| Dinner | 405 cal |
| Dessert | 155 cal |
| Bedtime snack | <u>100 cal</u> |
| | 1,280 cal |

**Sample Day**

| | | |
|---|---|---|
| Breakfast: | 2 low-fat pancakes, with butter and 0-calorie maple syrup | 160 cal |
| Midmorning snack | Hershey's Reese's Peanut Butter Wafer Bar | 100 cal |
| Lunch | Ham sandwich: 5 slices ham, 2 slices bread and 1 Tbs. mayo | 140 cal |
| Tea | 2 slices bread or toast with 1 Tbs. cream cheese or 2 Tbs. butter with sliced cucumber or lettuce | 100 cal |
| Dinner | Healthy Choice Chicken Teriyaki | 280 cal |
| | One-pound bag broccoli or cauliflower | 125 cal |
| Dessert | Silhouette Vanilla ice-cream sandwich | 130 cal |
| | Swiss Miss Hot Cocoa Mix, Diet w/ Calcium | 25 cal |
| Bedtime snack | Tea sandwich: 2 slices toast, 1Tbs. fat-free cream cheese with Walden Farms jelly or jam | 100 cal |
| Gold Coins | Snacks to quell hunger. Refer to choices on page 44 | <u>120 cal</u> |
| | | 1,280 cal |

## Calorie Outline and Sample Day
### 1,540 calorie outline — For the average American man

The average American man is 5 foot 9 inches tall. He should weigh 154 pounds and should consume 1,900 calories a day. I will keep him full on 1,540 calories a day (154 x 10 = 1,540 cal). He will be full and lose at the ideal rate of about a pound a week.

| | |
|---|---|
| Breakfast | 150 cal |
| Midmorning snack | 100 cal |
| Lunch | 280 cal |
| Gold coins | 130 cal |
| Tea sandwiches | 200 cal |
| Dinner | 580 cal |
| Dessert | 100 cal |
| | 1,540 cal |

### Sample Day

| | | |
|---|---|---|
| Breakfast | 2 low-fat pancakes, with butter and 0-calorie maple syrup | 150 cal |
| Midmorning snack | Hershey's York Peppermint Wafer Bar | 100 cal |
| Lunch | 2 ham sandwiches, each made with 5 slices ham, 2 slices bread and 1 Tbs. mayo | 280 cal |
| Tea | 2 tea sandwiches, each made with 2 slices bread toast with 1 Tbs. cream cheese and 1 Tbs. butter with sliced cucumber or lettuce | 200 cal |
| Dinner | Healthy Choice Chicken Teriyaki plus One-pound bag of FreshDirect mixed vegetables | 420 cal 160 cal |
| Dessert | Klondike Slim-a-Bear bar: | 100 cal |
| Gold coins | Snacks to quell hunger. Refer to choices on page 44 | 130 cal 1,540 cal |

**Festive Living for the Average American Woman**
1,650 Calories

The average American woman weighs about 154 pounds and should weigh about 128 pounds. After she has slimmed down to her proper weight, she can maintain it by being full on 13 calories per pound, about 1,650 calories.

| | | |
|---|---|---:|
| Breakfast | 2 low-fat pancakes with butter and syrup | 150 cal |
| | Black coffee or other no-cal drink | 0 cal |
| Midmorning Snack | Hostess 100-calorie 3-pack mini muffins | 100 cal |
| Tea sandwich | 2 slices bread, 2 Tbs. butter, or 1 Tbs. cream cheese or mayo, and sliced cucumber or lettuce leaves | 90 cal |
| Lunch | Ham sandwich: 5 ham, 2 slices bread and 1 Tbs. mayo | 140 cal |
| | No-calorie beverage | 0 cal |
| Afternoon snack | Cinnamon toast 2 slices bread, 2 Tbs. butter, 2 packets Splenda and a sprinkle of cinnamon | 90 cal |
| | No-calorie beverage | 0 cal |
| Dinner | Lean Cuisine Steak Tips Dijon | 280 cal |
| | *or* Healthy Choice French Bread Pizza | *350 cal* |
| | Side Salad* | 30 cal |
| | Popcorn – Orville Redenbacher's single serving Smart Pop mini-bag popcorn | 100 cal |
| Dessert | 1 package Jell-O Sugar-free Cook & Serve Chocolate pudding made with 1 cup water, 4 Tbs. Reddi-wip topping | 150 cal |
| Late-night snack | Tea sandwich: 2 slices toast, 1Tbs. fat-free cream cheese with Walden Farms jelly or jam | 100 cal |
| Gold Coins | Snacks to quell hunger. Refer to choices on page 44 | <u>90 cal</u> |
| | | 1,300 cal |

*The calories of the salad depend on how much lettuce is being used: 1 leaf is 1 calorie, 1 cup is 7 calories, 1 head of lettuce (5" in diameter) is 21 calories. A Side Salad is about 30 calories.

# Once You've Reached Your Ideal Weight

**Festive Living for the Average American Man**
2,000 Calories

The average American male should weigh about 154 pounds. Once he finishes slimming down to his ideal weight, staying full on 13 calories per pound will maintain that weight.

| | | |
|---|---|---|
| Breakfast | 2 low-fat pancakes with butter and syrup | 150 cal |
| | Black coffee or other no-cal drink | 0 cal |
| Midmorning Snack | Hostess 3-pack | 100 cal |
| Tea sandwich | 2 slices bread, 2 Tbs. butter, or 1 Tbs. cream cheese or 1 Tbs. mayo and cucumber slices or lettuce | 100 cal |
| Lunch | 2 ham sandwiches | 280 cal |
| | No-calorie beverage | 0 cal |
| | Mini-bag popcorn | 100 cal |
| Afternoon Snack | Cinnamon Toast | 90 cal |
| | 2 slices bread, 2 Tbs. butter, 2 packets Splenda and a sprinkle of cinnamon | |
| | No-calorie beverage | 0 cal |
| Dinner | Swansons Turkey Breast & Stuffing Dinner | 370 cal |
| | Side Salad | 30 cal |
| | Hostess 3-pack | 100 cal |
| | Popcorn – Pop Secret Light Butter | 280 cal |
| Dessert | 1 package Jell-O Sugar-free Cook & Serve Chocolate Pudding made with 1 cup water, 4 Tbs. Reddi-wip topping | 150 cal |
| Late-night snack | Tea sandwich: 2 slices bread, 2 Tbs. butter or 1 Tbs. cream cheese or 1 tsp mayo, and sliced cucumber or lettuce | 100 cal |
| Gold Coins | Snacks to quell hunger. Refer to choices on page 44 | <u>110 cal</u> |
| | | 1,990 cal |

## Sample Day at 1,000 Calories | EXAMPLE 1

**Breakfast**: Waffles and Syrup

| | |
|---|---:|
| 2 fat-free waffles | 160 cal |
| 2 Tbs. Promise Ultra | 10 cal |
| Walden Farms syrup | 0 cal |
| Black coffee w/ Splenda | <u>0 cal</u> |
| | **170 cal** |

**Lunch:** Grilled cheese

| | |
|---|---:|
| 2 slices Wonder Light bread | 80 cal |
| 2 slices Smart Beat cheese | 50 cal |
| 2 Tbs. Promise Ultra | 10 cal |
| 1/2 bag Steamfresh Broccoli and Red Peppers | 75 cal |
| Walden Farms dressing | <u>0 cal</u> |
| | **215 cal** |

**Snacks**

| | |
|---|---:|
| Hostess 3-Pack | 100 cal |
| Small bag of popcorn | <u>100 cal</u> |
| | **200 cal** |

**Dinner:** Boca Burger Dinner

| | |
|---|---:|
| 2 Boca Burgers | 140 cal |
| 2 light buns | 160 cal |
| Lettuce and tomato | <u>10 cal</u> |
| | **310 cal** |

| | |
|---|---:|
| **Dessert:** Chocolate VitaMuffin | **100 cal** |
| **Gold Coins:** Snacks to quell hunger. Refer to choices on page 44 | **5 cal** |
| **Total** | **1,000 cal** |

**Sample Day at 1,000 Calories** | **E X A M P L E  2**

**Breakfast:** Cinnamon Toast Muffin

| | |
|---|---:|
| Light English muffin | 90 cal |
| Cinnamon and brown sugar Splenda | 0 cal |
| 2 Tbs. Promise Ultra | 10 cal |
| Mini V8 Juice | <u>30 cal</u> |
| | **130 cal** |

**Lunch:** Soup and Salad with garlic bread

| | |
|---|---:|
| 1 can Progresso 50% Less Sodium Chicken Noodle Soup | 180 cal |
| Side Salad with Walden Farms Dressing | 30 cal |
| 2 slices Wonder Light bread | 80 cal |
| 2 Tbs. Promise Ultra | 10 cal |
| Garlic powder | <u>0 cal</u> |
| | **300 cal** |

**Snack**

| | |
|---|---:|
| Small bag  popcorn | **100 cal** |

**Dinner:** Hot Dog Dinner

| | |
|---|---:|
| 2 light hot dogs | 80 cal |
| 2 light hot dog buns | 160 cal |
| 2 tsp. no-sugar-added relish | 10 cal |
| 2 Tbs. ketchup | 28 cal |
| 1 bag Steamfresh broccoli | 90 cal |
| Walden Farms dressing | <u>0 cal</u> |
| | **368 cal** |

**Dessert**

| | |
|---|---:|
| 1 box Sugar-Free Jell-O | 40 cal |
| 4 Tbs. Cool Whip Lite | <u>50 cal</u> |
| | **90 cal** |

| | |
|---|---:|
| **Gold Coins:** Snacks to quell hunger. Refer to choices on page 44 | **12 cal** |

| | |
|---|---:|
| **Total** | **1,000 cal** |

## Sample Day at 1,000 Calories | EXAMPLE 3

**Breakfast:** Eggs and Hashbrowns

| | |
|---|---|
| 1 Ida-Toaster hashbrown | 110 cal |
| 4 oz. Southwestern Egg Beaters | 60 cal |
| Coffee with 1/4 cup skim milk | <u>20 cal</u> |
| | **190 cal** |

**Lunch:** Bologna Sandwich

| | |
|---|---|
| 2 slices Wonder Light bread | 80 cal |
| 2 slices fat-free bologna | 50 cal |
| 1 slice Smart Beat cheese | 25 cal |
| Mustard | 0 cal |
| Side Salad | <u>30 cal</u> |
| | **185 cal** |

**Snack:** Tea Sandwiches

| | |
|---|---|
| 2 slices Wonder Light bread | 80 cal |
| 1/2 cup sliced cucumbers | 8 cal |
| Walden Farms onion dill dip | <u>0 cal</u> |
| | **88 cal** |

**Dinner:** Italian Sausage with Noodles

| | |
|---|---|
| 1 package Shirataki fettuccini noodles | 40 cal |
| 1 Shady Brook Farms hot Italian sausage | 160 cal |
| 1 cup sliced onions and green peppers | 30 cal |
| 1 spray Pam | 5 cal |
| Walden Farms Italian Dressing | <u>0 cal</u> |
| | **235 cal** |

**Snack**

| | |
|---|---|
| 1 small bag Pepperidge Farm Chessmen cookies | **100 cal** |

**Dessert**

| | |
|---|---|
| 1 package Jell-O Sugar-Free Fat-Free Chocolate Pudding made w/ 1 cup water | 120 cal |
| 4 Tbs. Cool Whip Lite | 50 cal |
| Walden Farms Caramel and Chocolate Sauce | <u>0 cal</u> |
| | **170 cal** |

| | |
|---|---|
| **Gold Coins:** Snacks to quell hunger. Refer to choices on page 44 | **32 cal** |

| | |
|---|---|
| Total | **1,000 cal** |

## Sample Day at 1,000 Calories | EXAMPLE 4

### Breakfast
| | |
|---|---:|
| 2 low-fat pancakes | 140 cal |
| Walden Farms Pancake Syrup | 0 cal |
| Coffee with 2 Tbs. Land O'Lakes Fat-Free Half & Half and Splenda | <u>20 cal</u> |
| | **160 cal** |

### Lunch
| | |
|---|---:|
| 2 cups Progresso 99% fat-free minestrone soup: | 200 cal |
| 1 slice Wonder Light toast with garlic and 1 Tbs. Promise Ultra | <u>50 cal</u> |
| | **250 cal** |

### Snack
| | |
|---|---:|
| 2 wedges Laughing Cow light cheese | 70 cal |
| 1 medium apple | <u>70 cal</u> |
| | **140 cal** |

### Dinner
| | |
|---|---:|
| Smart Ones Chicken Parmigiana | 300 cal |
| Side Salad | <u>30 cal</u> |
| | **330 cal** |

### Dessert
| | |
|---|---:|
| Klondike Slim-a-Bear bar | **100 cal** |

**Gold Coins:** Snacks to quell hunger. Refer to choices on page 44     **20 cal**

| | |
|---|---:|
| Total | **1,000 cal** |

## Sample Day at 1,000 Calories | EXAMPLE 5

### Breakfast
| | |
|---|---|
| 4 oz. Egg Beaters, scrambled | 60 cal |
| 2 slices Jennie-O Extra-Lean Turkey Bacon | 40 cal |
| 2 pieces Wonder Light toast with Walden Farms jam | 80 cal |
| Coffee with 2 Tbs. Land O'Lakes Fat-Free Half & Half | 20 cal |
| | **200 cal** |

### Lunch
| | |
|---|---|
| Lean Cuisine Southwest-Style Chicken Panini | **280 cal** |

### Snack
| | |
|---|---|
| 100-calorie bag popcorn | 100 cal |
| Skinny Cow Low-Fat Fudge Pop Mini | 50 cal |
| | **150 cal** |

### Dinner
| | |
|---|---|
| Package of Shirataki noodles | 40 cal |
| 1 Cup Ragú Light pasta sauce | 120 cal |
| 4 oz. can of green beans | 40 cal |
| | **178 cal** |

### Dessert
| | |
|---|---|
| Boo's Brownie from page 83 | **125 cal** |

**Gold Coins:** Snacks to quell hunger. Refer to choices on page 44     **45 cal**

| Total | **1,000 cal** |
|---|---|

## Sample Day at 1,100 Calories | E X A M P L E  1

**Breakfast**

| | |
|---|---:|
| 1 light English muffin | 90 cal |
| Walden Farms jam | 0 cal |
| 4 oz. Kraft Fat-Free cottage cheese | <u>80 cal</u> |
| | **170 cal** |

**Lunch:** Open Face Tuna Sandwiches

| | |
|---|---:|
| 2 slices Wonder Light bread | 80 cal |
| 1 small can tuna in water | 70 cal |
| 2 Tbs. fat-free mayo | 20 cal |
| 2 sticks celery | 0 cal |
| 2 slices SmartBeat cheese | 50 cal |
| Crystal Light | <u>5 cal</u> |
| | **225 cal** |

**Dinner:** Noodles and Chili

| | |
|---|---:|
| 1 package Shirataki spaghetti noodles | 40 cal |
| 2 cups Hormel 99% Fat Free Chili | <u>400 cal</u> |
| | **440 cal** |

**Snack**

| | |
|---|---:|
| Hostess 3-Pack | **100 cal** |

**Dessert**

| | |
|---|---:|
| Chocolate VitaMuffin | **100 cal** |

**Gold Coins:** Snacks to quell hunger. Refer to choices on page 44    **65 cal**

| | |
|---|---:|
| Total | **1,100 cal** |

## Sample Day at 1,100 Calories | EXAMPLE 2

**Breakfast**

French Toast recipe from page 72                                          160 cal

Coffee with 2 Tbs. Land O'Lakes Fat-Free Half & Half          <u>20 cal</u>

**180 cal**

**Lunch:** Turkey & Cheese Sandwich

2 slices Wonder Light with 5 slices Hillshire Farms Deli-Select          170 cal
   smoked turkey breast and 2 slices Smart Beat

2 Kraft Twist-Ums string cheese                                          <u>120 cal</u>

**290 cal**

**Snack**

100-calorie bag popcorn                                                   100 cal

**Dinner**

Double Cheeseburger recipe from page 101                                  315 cal

**Dessert**

1/8 serving Boo's Cheesecake recipe from page 81                          138 cal

**Gold Coins:** Snacks to quell hunger. Refer to choices on page 44          42 cal

Total                                                                     **1,100 cal**

## Sample Day at 1,100 Calories  |  EXAMPLE 3

### Breakfast
| | |
|---|---|
| 1 light English muffin | 90 cal |
| 4 oz. Kraft's fat-free cottage cheese | 80 cal |
| | **170 cal** |

### Snack
| | |
|---|---|
| Kraft Twist-Ums string cheese | **60 cal** |

### Lunch: Salad with Chicken
| | |
|---|---|
| 1/2 cup Perdue Shortcuts Chicken | 90 cal |
| 1 large tomato, diced | 33 cal |
| 1 cucumber, diced | 45 cal |
| 2 cups lettuce | 12 cal |
| Walden Farms Sweet Onion salad dressing | 0 cal |
| | **180 cal** |

### Snack
| | |
|---|---|
| 100-calorie bag of popcorn | **100 cal** |

### Dinner
| | |
|---|---|
| 10 oz. bag broccoli spears | 90 cal |
| Lean Cuisine Cheese Ravioli | 240 cal |
| | **330 cal** |

### Dessert
| | |
|---|---|
| 20 oz. can Comstock no sugar added apple pie filling | 245 cal |
| 4 Tbs. Reddi wip Fat Free topping | 10 cal |
| | **255 cal** |

| | |
|---|---|
| **Gold Coins:** Snacks to quell hunger. Refer to choices on page 44 | **5 cal** |

| | |
|---|---|
| Total | **1,100 calories** |

**Sample Day at 1,100 Calories** |

**Breakfast:** Omelet

| | |
|---|---:|
| 6 oz. Egg Beaters | 60 cal |
| 2 slices Smart Beat cheese | 50 cal |
| 1/2 cup diced tomato | 16 cal |
| 1/2 cup diced broccoli | 15 cal |
| 1 slice Wonder Light bread | 40 cal |
| 1 Tbs. Promise Ultra | 5 cal |
| Black coffee with Splenda | <u>0 cal</u> |
| | **186 cal** |

**Snack**

| | |
|---|---:|
| Hostess 3-pack | **100 cal** |

**Lunch:** Chef Salad

| | |
|---|---:|
| 3 cups Romaine lettuce, shredded | 30 cal |
| 1/2 cup chopped tomato | 16 cal |
| 1/2 cup chopped cucumber | 8 cal |
| 3 slices Hillshire Farm Deli Select Baked Ham | 30 cal |
| 3 slices Hillshire Farm Deli Select Smoked Turkey | 30 cal |
| 1 oz. Kraft Natural Shredded fat-free cheddar | 45 cal |
| Unlimited Walden Farms dressing of choice | 0 cal |
| 1 toasted light English muffin with 2 Tbs. Promise Ultra | <u>100 cal</u> |
| | **259 cal** |

**Snack**

| | |
|---|---:|
| 1 Special-K waffle with 2 Tbs. Promise Ultra | 90 cal |
| Unlimited Walden Farms jam | <u>0 cal</u> |
| | **90 cal** |

**Dinner:** Pasta and Cheese

| | |
|---|---:|
| 2 bags Shirataki fettuccini noodles | 80 cal |
| 4 slices Smart Beat cheese | 100 cal |
| 1 oz. Kraft Natural Shredded fat-free Cheddar | 45 cal |
| 3 Tbs. Promise Ultra | 15 cal |
| 1 package frozen broccoli with Walden Farms dressing | <u>90 cal</u> |
| | **330 cal** |

**Dessert:** 1 package sugar-free fat-free chocolate pudding (made with 1 cup water)    **120 cal**

**Gold Coins:** Snacks to quell hunger. Refer to choices on page 44    **35 cal**

| | |
|---|---:|
| **Total** | **1,100 cal** |

**Sample Day at 1,100 Calories** | E X A M P L E  5

**Breakfast:** Pancakes & Sausage

| | |
|---|---:|
| 2 Aunt Jemima low-fat pancakes | 140 cal |
| 2 Tbs. Promise Ultra | 10 cal |
| Unlimited Walden Farms pancake syrup | 0 cal |
| 2 Healthy Choice breakfast sausages | 50 cal |
| Black coffee with splenda | <u>0 cal</u> |
| | **200 cal** |

**Snack:** Apple with Cheese

| | |
|---|---:|
| 1 medium apple | 70 cal |
| 2 wedges Laughing Cow light cheese | <u>70 cal</u> |
| | **140 cal** |

**Lunch:** Chicken Melt

| | |
|---|---:|
| 1/2 cup Perdue Shortcuts Chicken | 90 cal |
| 2 leafs of lettuce | 2 cal |
| 1 large slice tomato | 5 cal |
| 1 Tbs. Kraft fat-free mayo | 10 cal |
| 2 slices Smart Beat cheese | 50 cal |
| 2 slices Wonder Light bread, toasted | <u>80 cal</u> |
| | **267 cal** |

**Snack**

| | |
|---|---:|
| 100-calorie bag of popcorn | **100 cal** |

**Dinner:** Simple Lo Mein

| | |
|---|---:|
| 2 packages Shirataki noodles | 80 cal |
| 1-lb. bag broccoli and cauliflower | 120 cal |
| 3 Tbs. House of Tsang Stir-fry Sauce | <u>75 cal</u> |
| | **275 cal** |

**Dessert**

| | |
|---|---:|
| Klondike Slim-a-Bear bar | **100 cal** |

**Gold Coins:** Snacks to quell hunger. Refer to choices on page 44     **18 cal**

| | |
|---|---:|
| **Total** | **1,100 cal** |

## Sample Day at 1,200 Calories | EXAMPLE 1

### Breakfast
| | |
|---|---:|
| 2 light English muffin | 180 cal |
| 4 Tbs. Promise Ultra Fat-Free margarine | 20 cal |
| Walden Farms jam | 0 cal |
| Black coffee with Splenda | <u>0 cal</u> |
| | **200 cal** |

### Lunch
| | |
|---|---:|
| 1 can chicken noodle soup | 160 cal |
| 2 slices light toast | 0 cal |
| 2 Tbs. Promise Ultra Fat-Free Margarine | 10 cal |
| Side salad | 30 cal |
| Diet Sprite | <u>0 cal</u> |
| | **280 cal** |

### Afternoon Snack
| | |
|---|---:|
| Yoplait-Covered yogurt stick | **110 cal** |

### Dinner
| | |
|---|---:|
| Medium baked potato | 160 cal |
| 2 Tbs. Kraft Fat-Free sour cream | 29 cal |
| 1 oz. Kraft Fat-Free cheddar cheese | 5 cal |
| 1 Tbs. Compliments bacon bits | 30 cal |
| 1 Shady Brook Farms hot Italian sausage | 160 cal |
| 1/2 cup green beans | 20 cal |
| | **394 cal** |

### Dessert
| | |
|---|---:|
| 1 Sara Lee's Triple Chocolate Fudge Brownie Bites | **90 cal** |

### Nighttime Snack
| | |
|---|---:|
| 100-calorie bag of popcorn | **100 cal** |

| | |
|---|---:|
| **Gold Coins:** Snacks to quell hunger. Refer to choices on page 44 | **26 cal** |

| | |
|---|---:|
| **Total** | **1,200 cal** |

## Sample Day at 1,200 Calories | EXAMPLE 2

### Breakfast

| | |
|---|---:|
| 3 Special-K fat-free waffles | 240 cal |
| Walden Farms no-calorie syrup | 0 cal |
| Coffee with 2 Tbs. Land O'Lakes Fat-Free Half & Half | 20 cal |
| | **240 cal** |

### Lunch

| | |
|---|---:|
| 2 slices Wonder Light | 80 cal |
| 2 slices fat-free bologna | 50 cal |
| 2 slices Smart Beat | 50 cal |
| Mustard | 0 cal |
| 2 Kraft Twist-Ums string cheese | 120 cal |
| | **300 cal** |

### Snack

| | |
|---|---:|
| Good Humor fat-free ice cream sandwich | **160 cal** |

### Dinner

| | |
|---|---:|
| Shirataki noodles | 40 cal |
| 4 Tbs. House of Tsang Stir-fry Sauce | 100 cal |
| 2 cups sliced mushrooms | 30 cal |
| 1 cup broccoli | 52 cal |
| | **222 cal** |

### Dessert

| | |
|---|---:|
| 1/5 of David Glass the Incredible Delicious Reduced-Fat Chocolate Truffle Cake | **180 cal** |

**Gold Coins:** Snacks to quell hunger. Refer to choices on page 44     **98 cal**

| | |
|---|---:|
| Total | **1,200 cal** |

## Sample Day at 1,200 Calories | EXAMPLE 3

### Breakfast
| | |
|---|---:|
| 2 slices light bread, toasted | 80 cal |
| Walden Farms jam of choice | 0 cal |
| 3 Tbs. Walden Farms Creamy Peanut Spread | 0 cal |
| Dannon Light & Fit Nonfat Yogurt | 60 cal |
| | **140 cal** |

### Snack
| | |
|---|---:|
| Twix 100-calorie bar | **100 cal** |

### Lunch: Salad with Chicken
| | |
|---|---:|
| 1/2 cup Perdue Shortcuts Chicken | 90 cal |
| 2 Tbs. Kraft Non-Fat Mayo | 20 cal |
| 1/4 cup grapes, halved | 16 cal |
| 1/4 cup chopped celery | 4 cal |
| 2 cups lettuce | 12 cal |
| | **142 cal** |

### Snack
| | |
|---|---:|
| 100-calorie bag of Chex Mix | **100 cal** |

### Dinner:
| | |
|---|---:|
| 1 package Shirataki noodles | 40 cal |
| 1 Shady Brook Farms hot Italian sausage | 160 cal |
| 1 cup Ragú Light Pasta Sauce | 120 cal |
| 2 Tbs. Parmesan cheese | 20 cal |
| 1 package frozen broccoli | 90 cal |
| | **430 cal** |

### Dessert
| | |
|---|---:|
| Klondike Slim-a-Bear bar | **100 cal** |

### Midnight Snack
| | |
|---|---:|
| 100-calorie bag of M&Ms | **100 cal** |

| | |
|---|---:|
| **Gold Coins:** Snacks to quell hunger. Refer to choices on page 44 | **88 cal** |

| | |
|---|---:|
| Total | **1,200 cal** |

## Sample Day at 1,300 Calories | EXAMPLE 1

### Breakfast
| | |
|---|---|
| Light bagel | 110 cal |
| 2 Tbs. fat-free cream cheese | 30 cal |
| 6 oz. Dannon Light & Fit Nonfat yogurt | 60 cal |
| Black coffee | 0 cal |
| | **200 cal** |

### Midmorning Snack
| | |
|---|---|
| Kraft Twist-Ums String Cheese | **60 cal** |

### Lunch
| | |
|---|---|
| 2 slices Wonder Light bread | 80 cal |
| 5 slices ham | 50 cal |
| 1 slice Smart Beat American cheese | 25 cal |
| 2 Tbs. Kraft non-fat mayo | 20 cal |
| 1/2 bag broccoli & red peppers | 75 cal |
| Diet Coke | 0 cal |
| | **250 cal** |

### Afternoon Snack
| | |
|---|---|
| 100-calorie Hostess Snack | **100 cal** |

### Dinner
| | |
|---|---|
| 1 package Shiritaki noodles | 40 cal |
| 1 cup chicken breast | 230 cal |
| 2 oz. Kraft Shredded Fat-Free cheddar cheese | 90 cal |
| Walden Farms pasta sauce | 0 cal |
| | **360 cal** |

### Dessert
| | |
|---|---|
| Good Humor fat-free ice cream sandwich | **160 cal** |

### Nighttime Snack
| | |
|---|---|
| 2 slices Wonder Light bread with Walden Farms jam | 80 cal |
| Tea | 0 cal |
| | **80 cal** |

| | |
|---|---|
| **Gold Coins:** Snacks to quell hunger. Refer to choices on page 44 | **90 cal** |

| | |
|---|---|
| **Total** | **1,300 cal** |

**Sample Day at 1,300 Calories** | **EXAMPLE 2**

**Breakfast:** Egg & Cheese Muffin

| | |
|---|---:|
| 1 light English muffin, toasted | 90 cal |
| 2 oz. Egg Beaters with yolk | 40 cal |
| 1 slice Smartbeat fat-free American cheese | 25 cal |
| Black coffee with Splenda | 0 cal |
| | **155 cal** |

**Midmorning Snack:** Apple & Peanut Butter

| | |
|---|---:|
| 1 medium apple | 70 cal |
| 1 Tbs. Walden Farms Creamy Peanut Spread | 0 cal |
| | **70 cal** |

**Lunch:** Club Sandwich

| | |
|---|---:|
| 2 slices light bread | 80 cal |
| 2 slices Hillshire Farms ham | 20 cal |
| 2 slices Hillshire Farms turkey | 16 cal |
| 1 slice turkey bacon | 20 cal |
| 1/2 cup iceberg lettuce | 3 cal |
| 2 slices tomato | 10 cal |
| 2 Tbs. Kraft's fat-free mayo | 20 cal |
| 100-calorie pack Lorna Doone cookies | 100 cal |
| | **269 cal** |

**Tea Snack:** Tea & Cucumber Sandwich

| | |
|---|---:|
| 2 slices light bread with 2 Tbs. Promise Ultra Margarine | 90 cal |
| 6 slices cucumber | 6 cal |
| Tea, with or without Splenda | 0 cal |
| | **96 cal** |

**Dinner:** Boca Burgers, Vegetables & Dessert

| | |
|---|---:|
| 2 original Boca Burgers | 140 cal |
| 2 light hamburger buns | 160 cal |
| 2 cups iceberg lettuce | 12 cal |
| 2 slices tomato | 10 cal |
| Small can of green beans with Walden Farms 0-cal. dressing | 40 cal |
| Low-fat ice-cream sandwich | 100 cal |
| | **442 cal** |

| | |
|---|---:|
| **Bedtime Snack:** Boston's light mini-popcorn bag | **70 cal** |
| **Gold Coins:** Snacks to quell hunger. Refer to choices on page 44 | **198 cal** |
| **TOTAL** | **1,300 cal** |

**Sample Day at 1,300 Calories** | E X A M P L E  3

**Breakfast:** Sausage & Eggs with Cinnamon & Sugar Toast

| | |
|---|---|
| 4 oz. Egg Beaters | 40 cal |
| 2 Healthy Choice breakfast sausages | 57 cal |
| 2 slices light bread | 80 cal |
| 2 Tbs. fat-free margarine | 10 cal |
| Splenda & cinnamon | <u>0 cal</u> |
| | **187 cal** |

**Morning Snack**                                                         **130 cal**
Granola bar

**Lunch:** Grilled Cheese Sandwich with Tomato Soup

| | |
|---|---|
| 2 slices light bread | 80 cal |
| 2 slices fat-free American cheese | 50 cal |
| 100-calorie instant tomato soup | <u>100 cal</u> |
| | **230 cal** |

**Afternoon Snack:** Apple with Cheese

| | |
|---|---|
| 1 medium apple | 70 cal |
| 2 wedges Laughing Cow light cheese | <u>70 cal</u> |
| | **140 cal** |

**Dinner**                                                                **370 cal**
Healthy Choice Chicken Parmigiana with spaghetti

**Dessert:** 3 mini-Milky Way bars                                        **120 cal**

**Gold Coins:** Snacks to quell hunger. Refer to choices on page 44       **123 cal**

| | |
|---|---|
| Total | **1,300 cal** |

## Sample Day at 1,300 Calories | EXAMPLE 4

**Breakfast**                                                                    **170 cal**
    2 fat-free waffles w/ fat-free margarine & sugar-free maple syrup

**Midmorning Snack**
    2 slices light bread, toasted with Walden Farms jam          80 cal
    Mini V8 Juice                                                <u>40 cal</u>
                                                                 **120 cal**

**Lunch**
    2 slices light bread                                         80 cal
    5 slices turkey breast                                       40 cal
    1 slice fat-free American cheese                             25 cal
    1 Tbs. fat-free mayo                                         10 cal
    Salad with Walden Farms dressing                             30 cal
    2 mini Snickers                                              <u>80 cal</u>
                                                                 **265 cal**

**Afternoon Snack:** 100 calorie Hostess Pack                                     **100 cal**

**Dinner**                                                                        **350 cal**
    French Bread Weight Watchers Pizza
    1/2 cup canned French-cut green beans

**Dessert**                                                                       **120 cal**
    1 package Jell-O Sugar-Free Fat-Free Chocolate Pudding made w/ 1 cup water

**Bedtime Snack**                                                                 **100 cal**
    100 calorie mini popcorn bag

**Gold Coins:** Snacks to quell hunger. Refer to choices on page 44               **75 cal**

**Total**                                                                         **1,300 cal**

**Sample Day at 1,300 Calories**

**Breakfast:** Bagel!

| | |
|---|---:|
| 1 Weight Watcher's bagel | 150 cal |
| 2 Tbs. Philadelphia Fat Free Whipped Cream Cheese | 30 cal |
| Unlimited Walden Farms jam | 0 cal |
| Black coffee | <u>0 cal</u> |
| | **180 cal** |

**Midmorning Snack:** Apple with Cheese

| | |
|---|---:|
| 1 medium apple | 70 cal |
| 2 wedges Laughing Cow light cheese | <u>70 cal</u> |
| | **140 cal** |

**Lunch:** Corn Dogs

| | |
|---|---:|
| 2 Morningstar Corn Dogs with Walden Farms Barbecue Sauce | 300 cal |
| Salad with Walden Farms dressing | <u>30 cal</u> |
| | **330 cal** |

**Midafternoon snack**

| | |
|---|---:|
| 1 Boston's light mini-bag popcorn | **70 cal** |

**Dinner:** Spaghetti Bolognese

| | |
|---|---:|
| 2 packages Shiritaki spaghetti noodles | 80 cal |
| Unlimited Walden Farms tomato sauce | 0 cal |
| 2 cups Morningstar grillers recipe crumbles | <u>240 cal</u> |
| | **320 cal** |

**Desert**

| | |
|---|---:|
| Low-fat ice-cream sandwich | **100 cal** |

**Bedtime snack**

| | |
|---|---:|
| 1 Special-K waffle with Walden Farms jam | **80 cal** |

**Gold Coins:** Snacks to quell hunger. Refer to choices on page 44     **80 cal**

| | |
|---|---:|
| **Total** | **1,300 cal** |

## Sample Day at 1,400 Calories | E X A M P L E  1

**Breakfast:** Egg and Cheese Omlette

| | |
|---|---:|
| 6 oz. Egg Beaters | 60 cal |
| 3 slices fat-free American cheese | 75 cal |
| 1 slice toast with 1 Tbs. Promise Ultra | 45 cal |
| Black coffee with Splenda | 0 cal |
| | **180 cal** |

**Midmorning Snack:** Apple and Peanut Butter     **70 cal**

1 medium apple with 1 Tbs. Walden Farms Creamy Peanut Spread

**Lunch:** Tofu Stir-Fry

| | |
|---|---:|
| 1/2 package (158 g) Nasoya lite firm tofu | 80 cal |
| 1 package Bird's Eye Steamfresh broccoli | 120 cal |
| 2 Tbs. House of Tsang Classic Stir-Fry Sauce | 50 cal |
| | **250 cal** |

**Afternoon Snack:** Tea and Biscotti

| | |
|---|---:|
| Black tea (with or without Splenda) | 0 cal |
| 1 Nonni Biscotti | 110 cal |
| | **110 cal** |

**Dinner:** Fettuccini Alfredo with Mushrooms and "Chicken"

| | |
|---|---:|
| 2 packages Shirataki fettuccini | 80 cal |
| 1 package (8 oz) baby portabello mushrooms | 50 cal |
| Unlimited Walden Farms Alfredo sauce | 0 cal |
| 1 Quorn Naked Chik'n Cutlet | 80 cal |
| Side Salad with Walden Farms dressing | 30 cal |
| | **240 cal** |

**Dessert:**

| | |
|---|---:|
| 1 package Jell-O sugar-free cook & serve chocolate pudding (made with 2 cups skim milk) | **280 cal** |

**Bedtime Snack**

| | |
|---|---:|
| Boston's light mini-bag popcorn | 70 cal |
| 100 calorie 3 Musketeers Bar | 100 cal |
| | **170 cal** |

**Gold Coins:** Snacks to quell hunger. Refer to choices on page 44     **100 cal**

| | |
|---|---:|
| Total | **1,400 cal** |

## Sample Day at 1,400 Calories | **EXAMPLE 2**

**Breakfast**: Egg and Cheese Sandwich

| | |
|---|---:|
| 1 lite English muffin, toasted with 2 Tbs. Promise Ultra | 100 cal |
| 4 oz. Egg Beaters | 40 cal |
| 2 slices Smart Beat cheese | 50 cal |
| 1 Dannon Light & Fit Nonfat yogurt | <u>60 cal</u> |
| | **250 cal** |

**Snack**: Apple and Peanut Butter

| | |
|---|---:|
| 1 medium apple | 70 cal |
| 3 Tbs. Walden Farms Creamy Peanut Spread | <u>0 cal</u> |
| | **70 cal** |

**Lunch**: Chicken Caesar Salad

| | |
|---|---:|
| 1/2 cup Perdue Shortcuts Chicken | 90 cal |
| 3 cups Romaine lettuce, shredded | 30 cal |
| Walden Farms Caesar Dressing | 0 cal |
| 4 Tbs. grated Parmesan cheese | 40 cal |
| 2 slices Wonder Light, toasted | 80 cal |
| 2 Tbs. Promise Ultra | <u>10 cal</u> |
| | **250 cal** |

**Snack**

| | |
|---|---:|
| 100-calorie Hostess Pack | **100 cal** |

**Dinner**: Shrimp Alfredo

| | |
|---|---:|
| 2 packages Shirataki fettuccini | 80 cal |
| Unlimited Walden Farms alfredo sauce | 0 cal |
| 3 oz. shrimp | 84 cal |
| 1/2 bag broccoli and red peppers with Walden Farms dressing | <u>75 cal</u> |
| | **239 cal** |

**Dessert**

| | |
|---|---:|
| 1/2 pint Stonyfield Farms Frozen Yogurt | 200 cal |
| 4 Tbs. Reddi-wip | 30 cal |
| Walden Farms Caramel and Chocolate Sauce | <u>0 cal</u> |
| | **230 cal** |

**Late-Night Snack**

| | |
|---|---:|
| 100-calorie bag of popcorn | **100 cal** |

**Gold Coins**: Snacks to quell hunger. Refer to choices on page 44     **161 cal**

| | |
|---|---:|
| **Total** | **1,400 cal** |

## Sample Day at 1,600 Calories  |  **EXAMPLE 1**

### Breakfast
| | |
|---|---:|
| 3 Banquet Turkey sausages | 110 cal |
| 4 pieces of Wonder Light bread with Walden Farms jam | 160 cal |
| Mini V8 | <u>30 cal</u> |
| | **305 cal** |

### Midmorning Snack
| | |
|---|---:|
| Sugar-free Jell-O snack cup | **10 cal** |

### Lunch: Ham Sandwich
| | |
|---|---:|
| 5 slices Hilshire Farms ham, 2 pieces Wonder Light bread, 1 Tbs. Kraft fat-free mayo | 140 cal |
| Medium apple with Walden Farms Creamy Peanut Spread | <u>70 cal</u> |
| | **216 cal** |

### Snack
| | |
|---|---:|
| Snack-Away Yogurt Creme Oatmeal Cookie | 100 cal |
| 1 package Jet-Puffed ChocoMallows | <u>90 cal</u> |
| | **190 cal** |

### Dinner
| | |
|---|---:|
| Two servings of Hamburger Helper Microwave Singles Cheesy Lasagna | **420 cal** |

### Dessert
| | |
|---|---:|
| 3 mini-Milky Way bars | 120 cal |
| 1 Fun-Size Snickers | 70 cal |
| 2 packages 100-calorie Hostess Snacks | <u>200 cal</u> |
| | **390 cal** |

**Gold Coins:** Snacks to quell hunger. Refer to choices on page 44   **75 cal**

| | |
|---|---:|
| Total | **1,600 cal** |

# Sample Day at 1,600 Calories | EXAMPLE 2

## Breakfast
| | |
|---|---|
| 1 cup of scrambled Egg Beaters (southwestern flavor) | 120 cal |
| 3 Banquet Turkey sausages | 110 cal |
| 2 pieces of Wonder Light bread with Walden Farms jam | <u>80 cal</u> |
| | **220 cal** |

## Midmorning Snack
| | |
|---|---|
| 100-calorie bag of Smart Pop popcorn | 100 cal |
| Mini V8 | <u>30 cal</u> |
| | **130 cal** |

## Lunch: 2 Peanut Butter and Jelly Sandwiches
| | |
|---|---|
| 4 slices Wonder Light bread | 160 cal |
| 4 Tbs. Walden Farms Creamy Peanut Spread | 0 cal |
| Walden Farms Jam | <u>0 cal</u> |
| | **160 cal** |

## Snack:
| | |
|---|---|
| 100-calorie pack Goldfish (extra cheddar flavor) | 100 cal |
| 1 medium apple and a wedge of Laughing Cow cheese | <u>105 cal</u> |
| | **205 cal** |

## Dinner: Bacon Cheeseburgers
| | |
|---|---|
| 2 Boca Burgers (70 calories each) | 140 cal |
| 2 slices Smart Beat cheddar cheese (25 calories each) | 50 cal |
| 2 Light hamburger buns (80 calories each) | 160 cal |
| 4 Jenny O Lean Turkey Bacon Strips (20 calories per piece) | 80 cal |
| Small can of green beans | <u>30 cal</u> |
| | **460 cal** |

## Dessert
| | |
|---|---|
| 3 chocolate VitaMuffins (100 cal each) | **300 cal** |

**Gold Coins:** Snacks to quell hunger. Refer to choices on page 44     **125 cal**

---

**Total**     **1,600 cal**

**Sample Day at 1,600 Calories** | **EXAMPLE 3**

**Breakfast:** Peanut Butter Toast

| | |
|---|---|
| 3 pieces of Wonder Light bread, toasted | 120 cal |
| 4 Tbs. of Walden Farms Creamy Peanut Spread | 0 cal |
| | **120 cal** |

**Mid-morning Snack**

| | |
|---|---|
| 1 medium apple and Laughing Cow light cheese wedge | **130 cal** |

**Lunch:** Tuna Melt

| | |
|---|---|
| Small can of Bumble Bee tuna in water | 70 cal |
| 1 Tbs. Kraft fat-free mayo | 10 cal |
| 2 slices Wonder Light bread | 80 cal |
| 2 slices Smart Beat cheddar cheese | 50 cal |
| 100-calorie pack of Goldfish | 100 cal |
| | **310 cal** |

**Snacks for any time**

| | |
|---|---|
| 100-calorie Hostess Pack | 100 cal |
| Mini V8 | 30 cal |
| 1 Chiclet sugarless gum | 3 cal |
| | **133 cal** |

**Dinner**

| | |
|---|---|
| 2 servings Festive Chili (see recipe on page 97) | **560 cal** |

**Dessert**

| | |
|---|---|
| 1 package Jell-O Sugar-Free Fat-Free Chocolate Pudding made w/ 1 cup water with 4 Tbs. of Reddi-Whip | **150 cal** |

**Gold Coins:** Snacks to quell hunger. Refer to choices on page 44     **197 cal**

| | |
|---|---|
| Total | **1,600 cal** |

**Shocker 1:**
**Pasta and Cake**

| | |
|---|---:|
| 5 packages Shiritake Noodles with Tofu (40 calories each) | 200 cal |
| with unlimited Walden Farms Tomato or Alfredo sauce | |
| 10 @ 100-calorie packs of Hostess Mini Cupcakes (30 cakes!) | <u>1,000 cal</u> |
| **Total** | **1,200 cal** |

**Shocker 2:**
**Breakfast all Day**

| | |
|---|---:|
| 14 Kelloggs Special K 99% fat-free Waffle  (14 x 80 calories) | 1,120 cal |
| 16 Promise Fat-Free Margarine 5 cal/ Tbs.  (16 x 5 calories) | 80 cal |
| Unlimited Walden Farms maple syrup | <u>0 cal</u> |
| **Total:** | **1,200 cal** |

**Shocker 3:**
**Achin' for Bacon**

| | |
|---|---:|
| 8 Boo's BLT sandwiches each made of: | |
| 3 Jenny O Lean Turkey Bacon Strips (20 calories per piece) | 60 cal |
| Wonder Light White Bread 2 slices (40 calories per slice) | 80 cal |
| Kraft Mayonnaise dressing 2 Tbs. (10 calories) | 10 cal |
| 1 romaine lettuce leaf (1 calorie) | 1 cal |
| 1 slice medium tomato (4 calories) | <u>4 cal</u> |
| | 155 cal |
| | <u>x 8</u> |
| **Total:** | **1,240 cal** |

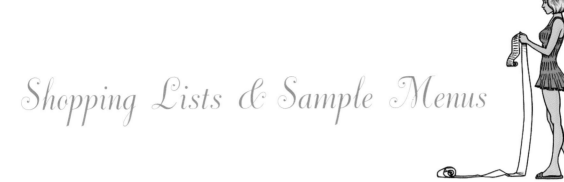

# CHAPTER 2

# Shopping Lists & Sample Menus

**Replace the high-calorie foods in your pantry and fridge with these:**

| | | Calories | |
|---|---|---:|---|
| a. | 40-calorie bread (light bread) | 40 | per slice |
| b. | Promise Ultra fat-free margarine | 5 | per Tbs. |
| c. | Kraft fat-free mayo | 10 | per Tbs. |
| d. | Sugar-free maple syrup | 0 | |
| e. | Fat-free cottage cheese | 10 | per Tbs. |
| f. | Reddi-wip Fat Free | 5 | per Tbs. |
| g. | Fat-free Italian dressing | 10 | per Tbs. |
| h. | Walden Farms Creamy Peanut Spread | 0 | |
| i. | Egg Beaters (or equiv.) | 10 | per oz. |
| j. | Laughing Cow light original cheese wedge | 35 | per wedge |
| k. | Hillshire Farms ham or turkey | 10 | ham |
| | | 8 | turkey |
| l. | Smartbeat Fat-free American cheese slice | 25 | each |
| m. | Small can Bumble Bee tuna in water | 70 | |
| n. | Generic sugar-free pudding | 120 | per box |
| p. | Pop Secret Butter Light Popcorn | 280 | per bag |
| q. | Fat-free cream cheese | 15 | per Tbs. |
| r. | Calorie-free Walden Farms jam with Splenda | 0 | |

*(Letters are referenced in the meal choices that follow)*

## Shopping List by Category:

### DAIRY

| | | Calories | |
|---|---|---|---|
| **n.** | Generic sugar-free pudding | 120 | per box |
| **b.** | Promise Ultra fat-free margarine | 5 | per Tbs. |
| **e.** | Fat-free cottage cheese | 10 | per Tbs. |
| **f.** | Reddi-wip Fat Free | 5 | per Tbs. |
| **i.** | Egg Beaters (or equiv.) | 10 | per ounce |
| **j.** | Laughing Cow light original cheese wedge | 35 | per wedge |
| **l.** | Smartbeat Fat-free American cheese slices | 25 | each |
| **q.** | Fat-free cream cheese | 15 | per Tbs. |

### MEAT

| | | | |
|---|---|---|---|
| **k.** | Hillshire Farms ham or turkey | 10 | ham |
| | | 8 | turkey |

### PANTRY

| | | | |
|---|---|---|---|
| **c.** | Kraft fat-free mayo | 10 | per Tbs. |
| **d.** | Sugar-free maple syrup | 0 | |
| **g.** | Fat-free Italian dressing | 10 | per Tbs. |
| **h.** | Walden Farms Creamy Peanut Spread | 0 | |
| **m.** | Small can Bumble Bee tuna in water | 70 | |
| **n.** | Generic sugar-free pudding | 120 | per box |
| **p.** | Pop Secret Popcorn Light butter popcorn | 280 | per bag |
| **r.** | Calorie-free Walden Farms jam with Splenda | 0 | |

### BREAD

| | | | |
|---|---|---|---|
| **a.** | 40-calorie bread (light bread) | 40 | per slice |

*(Letters are referenced in the meal choices that follow)*

**Sample menu choices**

*Letters refer to shopping list.*

## BREAKFAST CHOICES — approximately **150 calories**

| | |
|---|---|
| 2 fat-free waffles, with butter [b] and maple syrup [d] | 170 cal |
| 2 scrambled eggs (4 oz. Egg Beaters [i]) 2 slices turkey bacon, toast [a], 1 Tbs. butter [b] | 145 cal |
| Light English muffin with one wedge of cheese [j] and 1 Tbs. of butter [b] | 140 cal |
| 3 slices toast [a] with 2 Tbs. sugar-free jam and 3 Tbs. butter [b] | 135 cal |
| Cinnamon toast: [a] 3 slices of toast with 3 Tbs. butter [b] Sprinkle each slice with cinnamon and packets of sugar substitute. | 135 cal |
| Eggs Benedict: one poached egg, light English muffin, 1 Tbs. Boo's hollandaise sauce (sauce is made with 2 cups fat-free cottage cheese with 2 tsp. Durkee's butter extract), 1 slice Canadian bacon, 1 Tbs. butter [b] | 220 cal |
| French toast: 4 oz. Egg Beaters [i] and 2 slices white bread [a] with 2 Tbs. butter [b] and maple syrup [d] | 150 cal |
| 2 low-fat pancakes with 2 Tbs. butter [b] and maple syrup [d] | 150 cal |

## LUNCH CHOICES — approximately **150 calories**

| | |
|---|---|
| Ham sandwich<br>(5 slices ham [k], 2 slices bread [a] and 1 Tbs. mayo [c]) | 140 cal |
| Turkey sandwich<br>(5 slices turkey [k], 2 slices bread [a], 1 Tbs. mayo [c]) | 132 cal |
| Bologna sandwich (2 slices fat-free bologna, 2 slices bread [a],<br>lettuce, tomato and 1 Tbs. mayo [c]) | 135 cal |
| Peanut butter and jelly sandwich (2 Tbs. peanut butter [h]),<br>1 Tbs. calorie-free jelly [r], 2 slices bread [a]) | 80 cal |
| Medium apple and cheese wedge [j] | 140 cal |
| Tuna [m] with 1 Tbs. mayo [c], 1slice of toast [a], lettuce, tomato | 120 cal |
| Lipton Creamy Cup-A-Soup, 2 slices of toast [a], lettuce | 140 cal |
| Open-faced grilled-cheese sandwich<br>(2 slices cheese [l], 2 slices bread[a]) | 130 cal |

## DINNER CHOICES — approximately **400 calories** (with vegetable)

### Lean Cuisine (or equivalent)

| | |
|---|---|
| Lean Cuisine Steak Tips Dijon | 280 cal |
| Healthy Choice Oriental-style chicken (or equivalent) | 230 cal |
| Deluxe French Bread Pizza Weight Watchers (or equivalent) | 310 cal |
| Lean Cuisine Salisbury Steak | 280 cal |

### Boo's Dinners

| | |
|---|---|
| Egg Foo Yung (*see recipe on page 93*) | 200 cal |
| Two Boca burgers, 2 light hamburger buns | 300 cal |

*To make a filling meal and reach 400 cal. out of all of the above, add*:

| | |
|---|---|
| side salad with fat-free Italian dressing | 30 cal |
| or small can green beans | 40 cal |
| or brick of frozen broccoli spears | 90 cal |
| or bag of frozen broccoli, cauliflower, green beans, etc. | 100–150 cal |

## DESSERT CHOICES

| | |
|---|---|
| Chocolate pudding [n] with Reddi-wip Light [f] | 150 cal |
| Smart Pop microwave popcorn mini size – Orville Redenbacher | 100 cal |
| Sugar-free Jell-O with Reddi-wip Light [f] | 50 cal |
| Generic cereal bar or granola bar | 90 – 130cal |
| Low-fat ice-cream sandwich | 100 cal |
| Medium apple and cheese wedge [j] | 140 cal |
| Miniature Milky Way or Snickers | 40 cal |
| Fun-Size Snicker bar | 70 cal |
| Mini V8 juice | 30 cal |
| Boston's light mini-bag popcorn | 70 cal |
| Hostess 100-calorie Packs | 100 cal |

*Cupcakes, carrot cakes, blueberry, banana, or cinnamon coffee cake muffins*

| | |
|---|---|
| Frozen berries with Walden Farms Chocolate Syrup and Splenda | 70 cal |
| Fruit leather | 45 cal |
| Klondike Slim-a-Bear bars and sandwiches | 100 cal |

## TEA AND TOAST CHOICES

| | |
|---|---|
| 2 slices bread [a] or toast [a] (40 each) with 1 Tbs. cream cheese [q] (15 cal) and 1 Tbs. butter [b] (5 cal) | 100 cal |
| or: 2 Tbs. butter [b] and 2 Splenda packets and cinnamon | 90 cal |
| or: 2 Tbs. butter [b] and sliced cucumber or lettuce | 90 cal |
| or: 1 Tbs. jam [r] and 1 Tbs. butter [b] | 85 cal |
| or: 1 Tbs. cream cheese [q] and 1 Tbs. butter [b] and sliced cucumber or lettuce | 100 cal |

## GOLD COINS — approximately **100 calories**
*(Low-cal goodies to quell hunger pangs should they arise.)*

I plan my diet to include 100 calories of "gold coins." These "coins" are 100 calories per day of delicious tidbits that are between 1 and 10 calories apiece. The market is full of these "gold coins." My personal favorites are pretzel sticks at *2* calories each, Tic Tacs at 1 and *2*, Life Savers at 10, and mini jelly beans at 4 calories each. These "gold coins" cut off the hunger pangs at their inception. They are the other half of the Fullness Program. These 100 calories are as important to the program as the basic 13 calories times your ideal weight. Needless to say, I eat the pretzel sticks one at a time and suck the candies rather than chew them. This takes time and limits the intake of Gold Coins to about 100 calories a day.

| | |
|---|---|
| Tic Tac | 2 cal |
| Pretzel stick | 2 cal |
| Cinnamon red hot | 2 cal |
| Mini jelly bean | 4 cal |
| Chiclets Sugarless Gum | 3 cal |
| Gummy Bear | 6 cal |
| Life Savers | 10 cal |
| Stick of gum | 10 cal |
| Sugar-free Jell-O snack cup (really excellent and filling) | 10 cal |

# CHAPTER 3

# Shocking Calorie Savings

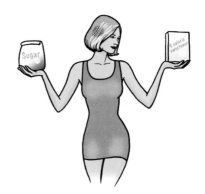

According to the USDA ERS research, daily calorie consumption per capita for the US was roughly broken down as such:

2005

| Meat, Eggs | Dairy | Fruit | Vegetables | Flour/Cereal | Added Fats | Added Sugars | Total |
|---|---|---|---|---|---|---|---|
| 463 calories/day | 279 calories/day | 80 calories/day | 125 calories/day | 611 calories/day | 644 calories/day | 477 calories/day | 2,681 calories/day |

If an individual replaced all of his/her added sugars with Splenda, he/she would be saving 477 calories a day, according to this research. It takes 3,500 calories burned to lose one pound of weight. Thus, just by switching to a no- calorie sweetener in foods and beverages, a person could lose almost a pound per week (3500/477 = 7.34, so he/she would lose a pound every 7.34 days). This means that in a month of using no-calorie sweeteners and products with no-calorie sweeteners, this lucky person would lose four pounds without having to change anything else about his or her diet.

Let's tackle data from the Per Capita Consumption Research, which gives annual consumption in pounds. According to this data from the USDA, in 2004 Americans consumed 33 pounds of eggs a year. According to thecaloriecounter.com, 1 cup of cooked, chopped egg (approximately 136 grams) has 211 calories. There are 453.59 grams to a pound, so in 2004 Americans consumed 33x453.59 = 14,968.47 grams of eggs. If 136 grams has 211 calories, then 1 gram has about 1.55 calories. So in 2004 Americans consumed about 23,223.14 calories from eggs.

Let's compare that to the amount of calories Americans would consume if they substituted Egg Beaters for all those eggs. According to the package, standard Egg Beaters have 30 calories per 61 grams. That means that 1 gram of Egg Beaters has about .49 calories. Taking the same data as before — that an average American eats 14,968.47 grams of eggs per year — that means that the Egg Beaters consumer would be eating 7,334.55 calories per year, in egg products, as opposed to the 23,223.14 calories that the individual using standard eggs would be consuming.

This means that by simply switching to Egg Beaters, the consumer is saving 15,888.59 calories a year or 1,324.05 calories per month.

**How about saving by switching to the 5-calorie butter?**
According to the USDA, Americans consume 9.9 pounds of butter per year. According to thecaloriecounter.com, 1 cup of butter, or 227 grams, has 1,628 calories. Since there are 453.59 grams to a pound, Americans in 2004 consumed 9.9x453.59 = 4,490.451 grams of butter. If 227 grams has 1,628 calories, then each gram has about 7.17 calories. So in one year on average, Americans consume 32,196.53 calories from butter.

Now, if the average American substituted Promise Ultra margarine for butter, his caloric savings would be huge. One tablespoon of Promise Ultra has 5 calories. One tablespoon is about 14.2 grams. So each gram of Promise Ultra has .35 calories. Using the same data as before, if the average American consumes 4,490.451 grams of butter per year, then the Promise Ultra consumer would eat 1,571.66 calories, as opposed to the 32,196.53 calories that the standard butter consumer would be ingesting in the year.

This data means that the Promise Ultra consumer is saving 30,624.87 calories per year, or 2,552.07 per month. In a year of embracing this negligible change, a dieter would lose almost 9 pounds, without having to change anything else about his or her diet.

# CHAPTER 4

# A Visit to the Market with Boo

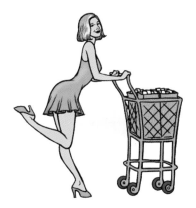

YOU BUY THE WONDER FOODS for my diet at the supermarket. I will take you around the store. We will start at the far end. The merchandisers know that the first item on most people's shopping list is milk. They make you go to the end of the store to get to the dairy section. They rely on your impulses to have you pick up additional items on the way. The first item in the dairy aisle is highly touted orange juice. I pass it by; I have better use for my calories. My daily multiple vitamin supplies all my vitamin C. The rest of the juice is mostly sucrose — sugar. If you love juice, Ocean Spray has a low-calorie line of juices sweetened with Splenda — quite delicious. Similar lines are coming out all the time.

My favorite milk is lactose-free, Lactaid fat-free milk. It is 10 calories an ounce, half the calories of regular milk. Its taste is like that of whole milk. Another option for skim milk with a richer taste is Skim Plus that is only 4 calories per ounce higher than regular skim milk. Land O'Lakes Fat Free Half & Half is sweet and creamy and only 10 calories per tablespoon. Use it liberally in your coffee and tea.

Next in the dairy section is butter. In this section my favorite wonder food is Promise Ultra fat-free margarine (5 calories per tablespoon as compared with regular Promise, which has 70 calories). It's not for use in cooking, but it spreads nicely on bread and vegetables and tastes delicious. For actual butter use Land O'Lakes Salted Whipped Light butter, which is 45 calories, as compared with Land O'Lakes 100-calorie butter. Still, it's no contest when compared with delicious fat-free Promise at **5 calories per tablespoon**. Reserve the whipped butter for cooking or when the butter flavor is critical. Philadelphia fat-free cream cheese is only 15 calories per tablespoon, as compared with the regular Philadelphia cream cheese at 45 calories per tablespoon, a wonder food no brainer.

Recently, tragedy has befallen my diet in the local supermarket. Extraordinary low-calorie products are being pulled off the shelves on nearly a weekly basis. The latest product on its way to being sacrificed is Promise Ultra Margarine, the remarkable 5-calorie butter substitute. It is a travesty that this incredible product is being removed from the local supermarket, presumably from lack of consumer interest. Promise Ultra is a true luxury item for the dieter — imagine, a product that truly tasted like butter for only 5 calories per tablespoon. That's a 95-calorie saving over regular butter, which is 100 calories per tablespoon. It has been estimated that the average American consumes 88 pounds of butter per year. If the average American simply switched to Promise Ultra, without changing anything else in his/her diet, he would save 88 pounds x 32 tablespoons per pound x 95 calories per tablespoon savings = 267,520 calories a year, which translates into 76.43 pounds per year (as 3,500 calories mean a pound of weight loss), or 1.47 pounds per week! It is truly a tragedy that a product that allows people to lose a pound and a half per week without having to make any kind of sacrifice will no longer be available to us locally.

Next to the butter section is the cheese. Regular cheese is high in calories with little filling power. A wonder drug exception is Twist-Ums by Kraft with cheddar cheese and mozzarella. The whole tasty stick is just 60 calories. fat-free and low-fat cheeses taste amazingly like their fatso brethren. They melt well and range in calories from 25 to 50 for the 2 percent singles — half the calories of the standard cheeses. Always buy fat-free or low-fat cheese.

Now we come to yogurts. Yogurts sweetened with Splenda or Nutrasweet are just as tasty as those sweetened with sugar. I'm always amazed that they still sell the sugary stuff. Why consume another 100 calories? Dannon offers a range of nonfat yogurts. Axelrod also has an excellent nonfat 90-calorie yogurt.  By the way, labels should not be scary. One friend shied away from low-calorie yogurt because it contained "chemicals." Dannon has a yogurt label that is mysterious until you analyze it. Aspartame is simply the technical name for Equal. Aspartame has been endorsed by the National Cancer Society as being absolutely pure. Modified food starch and pectin are natural and healthful. Whey protein concentrate is simply the protein of milk. Modified food starch is a low-calorie harmless version of good ole cornstarch. Whey is a natural byproduct of milk. (Remember Miss Muffet?) Citric acid is a harmless preservative found in a million products. Carrageenan and pectin are natural derivatives of seaweed and apple. Potassium sorbate is a harmless preservative used everywhere, and annatto is the natural yellow coloring used in Egg Beaters, etc. There are plenty of harmful chemicals in supermarket food, but I am extremely careful to recommend only the foods with the good ingredients.

Back to the dairy case where we now come to cottage cheese. Breakstone's fat-free, at 80 calories per serving/small container, is a third lower in calories than the 4 percent fat version — and the taste is good to excellent. Eaten with cucumber, or whatever, it would be impossible to tell which is the fat-free wonder drug cheese. Don't be a sucker. When sugar-free and fat-free taste as good or better than their fatty twins, reject the fat. Use the wonder food that didn't even exist a decade ago. Become slender while you are being self-indulgent.

Fat-free sour cream is another outstanding wonder food. Used with onion soup, it's the classic dip. Fat-free sour cream is about half the calories and tastier than the fatty version. I love to eat it by itself. I certainly use it wherever sour cream is indicated. Greg Northrop, my "sister" Rena's husband, loves tacos. We used to feel guilty when he topped the taco with a liberal dollop of regular sour cream. Now we feel gratified as we see him eat the same dish with fat-free sour cream. This section of the supermarket also features one of my bombshell secrets — Reddi-wip fat free topping. I love it on top of sugar-free Jell-O and all the other sugar-free puddings. There are only 10 calories in 1/2 cup of this formerly forbidden food.

Moving on, we come to the packaged meat department. Canadian bacon is my favorite. It is lean and 35 calories per ounce, as compared with 160 calories for regular bacon. The difference in calories is a measure of the difference in fat. Of the deli meats, I prefer Hillshire Farm Deli Select-Honey Ham, Smoked Turkey Breast and Baked Ham. They are from 97 to 99 percent fat-free and sliced so thin that they are only 20 calories per slice. Oscar Mayer Fat-free Bologna is only 25 calories per slice… Heaven. Oscar Mayer 98 percent fat-free hot dogs are 40 calories each, as compared with Oscar Mayer standard beef hot dogs at 180 calories each. The disparity of calories for similar-tasting meats makes it ludicrous to eat the standard product. I heartily recommend both the fat-free bologna and the fat-free hot dogs as basic wonder foods.

Shady Brook Farms has a sweet Italian and hot Italian sausage at 160 calories — a nice-sized link. This product has to be cooked thoroughly. It's the wonder drug sausage that I make part of my standard personal breakfast.

In the refrigerator case I recommend Perdue Breaded Chicken Breast Cutlets. Perdue also has chicken nuggets, which I recommend for adults as well as for kiddies.

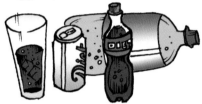

Next we visit the soda aisle. Soda made with sugar has been rightly called the worst killer in the supermarket. One brand has 150 calories in the 12-ounce can. A 20-ounce bottle of Classic Coca-Cola contains 17 teaspoons of sugar. Devastating. There is such a wide range of delicious diet sodas that it is criminal to drink sugared soda. The promoters of sugar-sweetened soda have to know that they are creating addicts. A drink of sugar water triggers the release of insulin. This is followed by a drop in blood sugar. This drop in blood sugar leads to immediate hunger pangs. The response to these pangs is to get another sugared drink or food. This lub-dub reaction is sharply defined by medical authorities as a primary cause of obesity and adult-onset diabetes, which is now sadly becoming common in children.

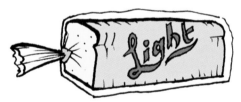

The bread aisle is next. Bread has always been 80 calories per slice. This has been an axiom forever, but the last few years have seen a wonder drug transformation. Wonder Light, Wonder Light Wheat, Wonder Light Italian are half the calories — just 40 per slice. They look the same and taste the same as the 80-calorie bread but are much richer in fiber. They are fundamental wonder foods. Even standard 90-calorie rye has its counterpart in 40-calorie light rye. Weight Watchers has a delicious deli-type 50-calorie-per-slice rye, which I recommend to you. Pepperidge Farm and others offer light and light-style bread in wheat, 7-grain, oatmeal, etc., and they keep coming out with more. Hot dog and hamburger buns are available at half the regular calories, and light English muffins are 90 calories instead of 140. Light breads are a revolutionary basis of my fullness program and in my opinion, a scientific breakthrough. It sickens me to see diet authorities torturing their clients by prescribing foods and calorically fattening bread and other foods when low-calorie substitutes are available on every grocer's shelf.

We are now at the ice-cream freezer. Premium ice creams, such as Häagen Dazs and Ben and Jerry's, run about 350 calories per half-cup — half the volume of your fist. Who can ever stop at only a half-cup? The equivalent fat-free is less than a third the calories — about 100. I find it even tastier because I have become unused to fat. I also enjoy Good Humor Fat-free Ice Cream Sandwiches at 160 calories and Yoplait coated yogurt sticks at 110.

As for frozen desserts, I favor the Weight Watchers Smart Ones line at around 150 calories, including a 200-calorie brownie. I disapprove of other famous desserts, such as Mrs. Smith's apple pie. They are high in calories for the taste and fillingness they offer.

Next come the frozen potatoes. Ore-Ida Toaster Hash Browns, one of my wonder drug favorites, are 110 calories per square. Very satisfying. I feature these at my dinners several times a month.

In the same freezer section are the frozen breakfast items. My favorite is Kellogg's Special K 99% fat-free waffles at 80 calories each. Add 5-calorie Promise margarine and 0-calorie Walden Farms maple syrup to create my wonder drug "belly-buster" breakfast. Also among my top recommendations are Weight Watchers Smart Ones, an excellent English muffin sandwich patterned after McDonald's Egg McMuffin, only 200 calories, excellent. A wonder drug staple, also found in the freezer breakfast section, is my "must have" Egg Beaters, now in three great flavors. Mixed into this section are Sara Lee's portion-controlled Triple Chocolate Fudge Brownie Bites — 90 calories a piece. A triumph in this department is Belgian mini éclairs by Delizza — 46 calories a piece. I serve these for dessert at least once a month. Also mixed in this area is the whipped topping I raved about previously, fat-free Reddi-wip.

TURN THE CORNER and we come to frozen dinners. They run the gamut from undesirable to superb. One doesn't have to be a rocket scientist to see that Banquet, Boston Market, and Marie Callender are loaded with sodium, calories, and fat. Their labels are all too specific. For your sake and your family's sake, read labels. Tiny local frozen-food manufactures may fudge on labeling calories and sodium — if they print them at all. They are too small for competitors to analyze and report. Major food producers can take no such chance. Their competitors are on the lookout for inaccuracies in their labeling and are eager to report them to the FDA. It is not idealism that keeps these producers honest. It is fear that they will be reported if they waver from the truth. The bottom line, though, is that we consumers are the beneficiaries. The labels on the frozen dinners of the major brands are accurate.

Along with reading the labels that scream of salt and fat and high-caloric content, it is pure delight to read the labels of my favorite wonder drug frozen dinners. They are the jewels in the crown of wonder foods. I'm just a bit envious of all you lucky people who are given these precious gifts of labeled, delicious, low-calorie gourmet dinners. I remember, with a touch of bitterness, the years when frozen dinners were called TV dinners — they were full of fat. What is worse, they had no indication of their calorie content. It was such a hassle to try to figure them out that the frozen dinner was anathema to me. I can't speak too critically of the old TV dinners. Similarly, I can't speak too highly of the new frozen dinners. Not one but three major firms turn out low-calorie, delicious dinners in an incredible variety. Healthy Choice is the best on sodium, but Lean Cuisine and Weight Watchers Smart Ones are equally superb. **Any of these low-calorie entrees can be turned into one of my Festive dinners by serving it with a brick of frozen vegetables. After microwaving the vegetables, make them sinfully rich by adding either Promise Ultra Fat-Free margarine or Molly McButter Cheese-Flavor Sprinkles or one of the creamy no-calorie dressings.** We elaborate on these special dinners in my recipe section. They are fast, filling, with clearly defined calorie content.

Next we come to the cookie aisle. Low-fat or no-fat diet crackers and cookies are a gyp. In these sugar-free products the manufacturers have taken the sugar out but replaced it with equal calories of maltodextrin. They are really no different in calories from the regular products. This also applies to baked versus fried potato chips.

In the soup department I enjoy Campbell's Double Noodle Soup. I add a 9-ounce brick of frozen cauliflower plus some water to make a Festive stew. It takes forever to eat and is thoroughly enjoyable. In the same category is Manhattan clam chowder plus cauliflower for a belly-buster stew for less than 250 calories. Progresso's Hearty Penne in Chicken Broth plus a 16-ounce can of green beans creates a luscious meal under 280 calories. Ditto for other combinations of soups and vegetables. This combo of soup and vegetable is a continuous wonder to me as one of the basis of my fullness program. The other evening I toasted a slice of Wonder Light Italian bread, topped it with a slice of two-percent Swiss cheese, and broiled this until the cheese melted. This I cut up and added to one can of Progresso French Onion soup. My husband and I shared and enjoyed this 200-calorie appetizer.

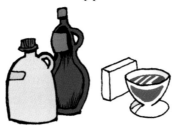

On to the syrups. These used to be my personal downfalls. I could eat pancakes and syrup forever. The skimpiest serving of pancake syrup is two ounces. I could easily pour double that onto my waffles. At 450 calories, the syrup alone was a big chunk of my daily calories. Imagine my delight at the development of a number of wonder drug low, or no-calorie maple syrups. I especially recommend Mrs. Butterworth and Walden Farms.

My favorite sugar-free pudding is chocolate. I make it with one cup of water so that it comes out like hot fudge. Delicious, 30 calories instead of 100. In the same section is the wonder food that is my personal secret weapon. Sugar-free Jell-O has no downside. It can be served by itself or with fruit or with whipped cream, etc. Even when Jell-O was 80 calories a serving, it was still a favorite among dieters. Cottage cheese and Jell-O plates were the staples of old-fashioned, pre-wonder drug diets. Imagine my joy with the development of sugar-free Jell-O — one-eighth the calories of its fattening twin. Sugar-free Jell-O is a must-have staple for your pantry.

The next aisle features protein extenders for family meals. I prepare Hamburger Helper with lean ground beef and Tuna Helper with tuna packed in water. I have friends who use these extenders several times a week. They find them invaluable. My household consists of my husband and me, so I rarely have use for them. For the standard American family of four or five, a family on the go and on a budget, these extenders are valuable staples. Other good ready-made, calorie-controlled and portion-controlled family dinners can be found back in the freezer section, such as the Lean Cuisine Skillet line. There is no downside to these products.

FYI: Always buy canned fruit packed in water. Sugar-free and low-sugar jams are obvious calorie savers. I recommend Peanut Wonder peanut butter at 100 calories instead of over 190. To save even more calories try Walden Farms Creamy Peanut Spread — 0 calories.

Regular beer is 160 calories as compared to 110 for light. Near beer is 70 calories. An ounce of liquor is 100 calories. Since an ounce is 2 tablespoons, a jigger of alcohol is 150 calories. Wine is basically 25 calories an ounce.

WE HAVE NOW COME FULL CIRCLE to the front of the store, where the produce is kept. Lettuce and popcorn provide your basic bulk. Your ideal is to focus on low-calorie vegetables, like string beans, cauliflower, broccoli, brussels sprouts, mushrooms, bean sprouts, peppers, celery, and spinach. A basic vegetable for my program is the string bean. I feel that it has every merit, but I am not as fanatical about it as a friend of mine. She has string beans at almost every dinner. She attributes her strength and health to her focus on this basic vegetable. She prides herself on making her vegetables even more delicious by smothering them in 5-calorie Promise Ultra margarine or Heinz fat-free gravy at 10 calories per ounce. Whether you are a moderate as I am or an extremist as she is, do make string beans a cornerstone vegetable of your menu. Be judicious in your use of the higher-calorie vegetables such as peas, lima beans, corn, carrots, and potatoes. Baked potatoes are 34 calories per ounce. Add the standard butter or other toppings, and the calories go off the chart. With the dressings on my shopping list, they can be acceptable because they are so filling.

I use my salad dressings for flavoring much more than salad. I use them as garnish for one vegetable after another. It's silly to let the name "salad dressing" force you to limit their use to salad. I use them for vegetables and on broiled meat, poultry, and fish. When I am out, if my diet dressings are not available, I choose oil and vinegar. I minimize the oil. One tablespoon of oil is 120 calories, and the flavor of the salad dressing has very little to do with the oil. At times, the oil actually detracts from the taste.

The dressings I chose to put on my shopping list contain harmless cellulose to thicken them, and they taste better than the high-calorie ones. I love the creamy fat-free Ranch, Caesar, Catalina, and Thousand Islands, which are only 35 or 40 calories per tablespoon, as compared with double the calories in the regular dressings. Fat-free Zesty Italian by Kraft is only 15 calories per tablespoon. I have stretched this dressing with vinegar and water, and it still retains its flavor. Some of the Walden Farms line are calorie-free.

Oddly enough, this produce area is where you find refrigerated tofu items. The winner in this category is the Shirataki noodle. It comes in a fettuccini style or spaghetti style. I am so greatly impressed with this product that I have devoted a whole chapter to this awesome product (*see Use Your Noodle, page 111*). A one-cup serving is 40 calories, as compared to 210 calories for regular wheat pasta or rice. I talk of the revolution in basic foods with 40-calorie bread, as opposed to 80. The Shirataki ratio is 40 to 210, or less than one-fifth. The equivalent of this wonder drug ratio would be to have a standard slice of bread at 14 calories instead of 80 for the regular and 40 for the light.

When science creates a new wonder drug, the discovery causes a momentary sensation. When Salk discovered his vaccine, the church bells around the world rang in celebration of the end of polio. Soon after, the discovery becomes just another fact of history. We tend to forget that there ever was a plague that crippled and killed tens of millions of people. I expect this to happen to our new wonder foods. Soon people will forget the dark ages of food in the past. They will forget that everyone knew that obesity was spreading dangerously, that mothers searched the food counters looking for nourishment that would keep the family trim. They looked at everything available, but nothing helped. There wasn't a calorie indicator on can or frozen package or, for that matter, on any food. Portion control was unheard of in the supermarket. The poor mother floundered through the various sections of the store finally seizing upon something to feed her family. The sense of helplessness in fighting obesity pervaded the atmosphere. I personally tried to calculate calories and weight and portion control, and it was no go. We were as helpless in fighting obesity before the new wonder foods as the poor mother was in fighting polio before the vaccine. There simply were no low-calorie, filling, tasty foods.

As dozens of other new wonder foods (including my forthcoming bar and shake) start to reverse the plague of obesity, there may be momentary rejoicing. Then, given human nature, everyone will forget that there ever was a time when obesity threatened the existence of humanity. They won't be able to imagine the helplessness of shopping for healthful foods when such foods just didn't exist. They will assume that any homemaker could always go to the market and choose among scores of chef-created, portion-controlled, delicious, moderately priced, low-calorie wonder foods. The wonder food will be just another fact of society, like the polio vaccine and streptomycin. The comforting fact is that at that time, the trend toward obesity will be reversed and slenderness will be the norm.

# FYI: PORTIONS AND CALORIES

A slice of bread is about one ounce. Every slice of standard bread is 80 calories. A bagel is the same 80 calories per ounce, but bagels are about 4–5 ounces. Cakes and muffins are 100 calories per ounce.

Regular butter is a killer. The tip of your thumb equals 1 tablespoon (100 calories). The tip of your pinkie equals 1 teaspoon. Even that tiny amount costs you 33 calories. Be sure to use my low-calorie alternatives.

A cup of cooked rice forms a ball the size of a baseball. It totals 210 calories. Ditto for pasta. Shirataki tofu noodles come in at a marvelous 40 calories. Shirataki noodles without the added tofu are even lower in calories. Ten calories per three-ounce portion. The five-portion package comes to only 50 calories.

Standard entrées are three ounces of cooked meat, the size of a deck of cards. Beef is 75 calories per ounce. Cooked hamburger is 70 calories per ounce. Chicken is 55 calories an ounce. Fish and shrimp are a caloric bargain at 35 calories an ounce.

My blockbuster classics, such as Renaissance, Walden Farms, and other no-cal jams, weigh in at zero, as compared with the usual 50 calories per tablespoon. My creamy salad dressing is zero instead of 140 calories. My pancake syrup is zero instead of 220.

Chips are 140 to 160 calories per ounce. Hard candy is a hefty 100 to 125 calories per ounce.

# CHAPTER 5

# The New Wonder Foods

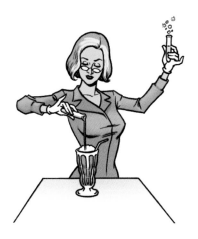

THE NEW FOODS developed over the past decade are as earthshaking in their power to overcome obesity as the wonder drugs were to overcome the illnesses they addressed. Before there was streptomycin, tuberculosis was a sentence of death. Now our kids hardly know the word tuberculosis. Before the Salk vaccine, even a president of the United States, Franklin Delano Roosevelt, became unable to walk, because there was no cure for polio. Now polio is just a bad memory.

I've been using the term "wonder drug." A wonder drug is "an agency, medical or other, that prevents or nullifies the destructiveness of what had been a major disease or deficiency." The new foods that provide tastes of sweetness and fat with minimal calories are as much wonder drugs as are penicillin, the Salk vaccine, etc.

Before the creation of the new foods, obesity was a hopeless condition. Most foods worth eating were loaded with sugar and fat. The foods that were low-calorie were considered rabbit food and inedible for any extended period of time. The authorities now agree that none of those old diets did work or could work. My new plan is so effective because it is based on the wonder foods, such as new sweeteners with low – no calories and fats with low – no calories. We now have a whole buffet table of rich foods that are so low in calories that you lose weight while eating "Festive meals."

In 2004 the UN pronounced obesity as the worst killer facing humanity. Equally stunning is the UN announcement that the plague is increasing in virulence and that there is no help in sight. We alone offer a solution in delicious, wonder food Festive meals.

My own dieting history began in the dark days before there were wonder foods. When I began dieting, losing weight was an agonizing, hopeless process, as it is for everyone today. Like the rest of the world, I tried the standard diets with the standard

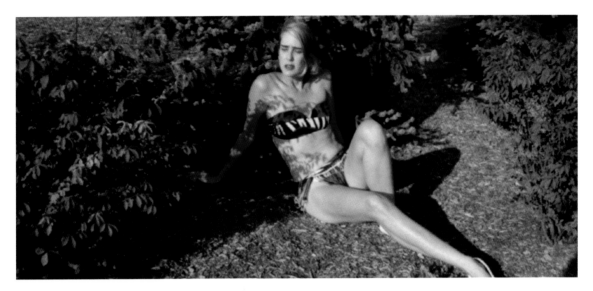

yo-yo of weight loss and weight regain. Everyone in my family had clothes ranging from "my sexy clothes" to "my fat clothes." Finally, my weight reached a point where my next fat clothes would be a size 18. I swore that I would never be an 18. I would rather spend my life hungry, subsisting on rabbit food. For reasons of vanity and health, I swore that I would spend my life as a size six.

I have my normal share of human failings, but I have one real virtue. I am strong-willed. I lived on celery and carrots and skim milk. I smiled grimly but refused to touch my slice of cake at the birthday parties. But I did remain a size six.

All this time, I haunted the supermarkets. I had to believe that there was a wonder drug, some food that would make my low-calorie life bearable. My first wonder food discovery was bread called "Less." It had half the calories of regular bread and tasted good. Suddenly I could eat two slices of bread for the calories of one. About the same time, Egg Beaters came out. At that time, they were tasteless, but I choked them down as a low-calorie source of protein. Then I was inspired to look at the diabetic section. Here I found foods made by Featherweight and Estee. I remember my nervousness at eating these foods meant for people with diabetes. Nevertheless, I experimented with them and soon added sugarless low- calorie pudding, gelatin, jelly and salad dressing to my meals. It was still grim going. I felt as if I were growing rabbit ears.

I tell of the odyssey of creating my program, shake and bar in my address to the doctors and nutritionists at Cornell. In short, my friends and I devoted years of time and tons of money to create this fullness program. We enlisted the help of university technicians and top food scientists from around the world. **The culmination of our work and dreams came in 2002. The US government formally recognized our program and awarded us a coveted patent for our shake and bar creations.** This is a most unusual commendation. We are gratified beyond words that our efforts have achieved such recognition.

Major inventions come in groups. The automobile, telephone and airplane were invented simultaneously in different countries by different people. One wonder drug food seemed to spark other wonder drug foods. In the past I had no choice but to eat tons of high-calorie sugar. It is hard to believe now, but I could find absolutely no sugar substitute that I could use. Saccharine, at that time, left a bitter aftertaste, and there were scary rumors about its causing cancer in rats. Cyclamates might well have been the answer, but then our government banned them. Finally, I contacted friends in Canada who got me cyclamates, which were available there. It was a laborious, expensive undertaking to get a sugar substitute. This experience is but a bad memory now. Today I can choose among half a dozen wonder drug sweeteners.

Once a few wonder drug products appeared on the market, the major food companies joined the parade. Suddenly the stores were full of wonder foods. The no-no foods that were "a moment on your lips and forever on your hips" were transformed into fat-fighting slenderizers. There was 40-calorie bread and 45-calorie butter. These two items are a revolution in themselves. Substituting them for the bread and butter you are now using would save you at least 6,000 calories a month — at least a pound and a half of weight. How nutritionists can work with overweight adults and youngsters and ignore this godsend is beyond me. Doctors love me. Every doctor who has read my book has given me hearty thumbs up. On the other hand, every nutritionist to whom I've shown my text has reacted with panicky hostility. How can they charge their impressive fees for their nutritional advice if I point out an easy delicious solution to obesity in the corner grocery store?

Bread and butter were just the beginning. There was 10-calorie mayonnaise, 25-calorie sour cream, 15-calorie cream cheese, zero-calorie salad dressing and 20-calorie gravy. The no-no foods that caused the bulge were now slenderizers. Low-calorie chocolate mousse, cheesecake, puddings and whipped cream now slimmed you down. The day of the wonder food had dawned. The new wonder foods offered endless possibilities for fulfilling the dream of our Festive diet of delicious foods that cause you to lose weight. I now had the panacea for the disease of obesity. With the appearance of the wonder foods, it would seem that we were at the end of the Dark Ages of the hunger diets that had failed. We were ready for the wonder drug Festive foods that would make us slim forever. But the fates had set forth another hurdle.

Medical and nutrition authorities had always agreed that weight was directly proportional to caloric intake. If you ate more calories than your body burned, your body would store these calories as fat. The couch potato eats chips, which the body turns into a spare tire. If the couch potato put away the chips and ate fewer calories, his body would have to burn the fat and so the spare tire would go.

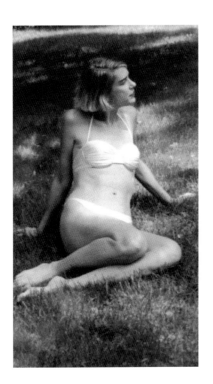

The fact that weight loss and weight gain depend on calories was never questioned — until Dr. Atkins. In 1970 my mother began to travel weekly from our home in Darien, Connecticut, to see a diet doctor in New York. Dr. Atkins told her that she could eat all the calories she wanted and would lose weight permanently if she avoided carbs. Calories were irrelevant. The only villain was the carbohydrate. My mother and one of my brothers were delighted with a diet that let them eat all the calories they wanted. They yo-yoed up and down on the Atkins diet for years. Just at the time that I formalized my program and the wonder drug of new foods was available, the Atkins mania exploded. He sold 15 million books; his apostles sold an additional like number. Calories were forgotten, and the only criterion for weight loss was "low carb." Thirty-five hundred items in the supermarket bore the red A for Atkins and/or the yellow "low carb" label. The *New York Times* began to give him credence. Other diet programs were quashed. When I tried to spread the word about my fullness program, I was met with a single response, "Is your program low-carb?"

During the hysteria Atkins was sacrosanct. Mayor Michael Bloomberg of New York City got into trouble by calling him "fat." When the highly respected Dr. Ornish challenged Atkins by saying that Atkins had never produced any scientific evidence for his program, Ornish was brushed aside. When Americans become fanatics, reason disappears. There were some medical voices that talked with horror about the damage to the liver, heart, etc., that could result from a diet of fat and protein. These voices were also brushed aside. Finally, the bubble burst. Starting in 2004, the Atkins' company lost tens of millions of dollars. Now that Atkins has died and his craze is old news, sanity is returning to the field of nutrition.

Our government for the umpteenth time announced this year that there is only one basis for obesity or for weight loss: eating more calories than you burn results in obesity; eating fewer calories than you burn results in weight loss. We are back to the simple fact that has been an axiom of medicine and nutrition from the beginning. Weight loss depends on eating low-calorie foods. Now that there are the new wonder low-calorie foods that are delicious, let's waste no more time. The obesity indicators are going through the ceiling. The cost to our nation of obesity is $117 billion this year, and it is skyrocketing. Let us confront the epidemic. The longest journey begins with a single step. Your job is to make yourself the svelte, lovely creature you were meant to be. Use the wonder foods science has given us. Plunge into my fullness program of rich low-calorie Festive meals. Be slender for life.

I want you to replicate in your life the odyssey of the lives of me and my sisters. What took me more than a decade to achieve, you can do in a day. The best way to begin our fullness program is to begin. Start our slenderizing program with a day of Festive meals. For breakfast slather our waffles with our butter and our jam, jelly, or our syrup. Dinner can be hot dogs and sauerkraut or our quiche for two.

At the same time, police your pantry, refrigerator and freezer. Replace your fatty bad foods with their slender twins. I've mentioned that the substitution of our light bread and our light butter for the standard products will mean a huge calorie savings — easily saving more than 6,000 calories — or a pound and a half a month. We are cautious about beginning too drastically. Our savings were calculated on substituting 45-calorie-per-tablespoon Land O'Lakes light whipped butter for 100-calorie-per-table-spoon Land O'Lakes regular butter. For those of you who are serious about a jump start toward slenderness, I want you to use the five-calorie-per-tablespoon Promise Ultra fat free instead of the 45-calorie Land O'Lakes light whipped butter. We use it for everything except cooking.

The calorie savings of using my basic products in place of the fatty ones are impressive. Even more impressive are the savings on foods in areas we don't consider staples. Who considers mayonnaise an important factor in slenderness? The 100 calories per tablespoon of ordinary Kraft mayonnaise seems trivial. Think, however, of tuna, potato, egg, chicken, and almost every other salad. Mayonnaise is the basic binder. At 10 calories per tablespoon for Kraft fat-free mayonnaise, or Hellman's 20-calorie per tablespoon, compared with 100-calorie-per-tablespoon Kraft or Hellman's, the caloric savings are obvious.

An equally important factor is the feeling of fullness my plan offers. As you use the full fat mayonnaise, you consciously or unconsciously hold back on the amount you use, because you know it's so fattening. With slenderizing mayonnaise, you feel full because you lavishly enrich your salads, since the mayonnaise is so low calorically. The bear is a vivid example of how nature makes us slender as we are full and how nature triggers fat storage and obesity with our feelings of hunger. (*See my address at Cornell on page 151.*)

What is true about mayonnaise applies equally to sour cream, cream cheese, gravy, salad dressing, jelly, and pancake syrup. Each of these condiments warrants a special description, which I will offer later. Exploring these new foods will be a culinary adventure. The points of reference about food that have governed you your whole life will be reversed. The once forbidden foods that are full of sugar and fat will now be low-calorie treats. The sour cream and gravy that made you fat in the past will now make you look like a pinup.

Conditioning can be a powerful force. For example, we are conditioned through experience that fire burns. If an inventor came up with cool flames, we would still be fearful of putting our hands into the "blaze." We could see by the thermometer that the "blaze" was at 70 degrees. Our intellects tell us that putting our hands into the blaze would be a completely positive experience. Our conditioning, however, is such that no matter what the thermometer said, we would hesitate to put our hand into the "blaze."

As I study the power of conditioning, I recall my own experiences. I knew every food and every calorie. Intellectually I knew that the foods I was eating would have to keep me slender because they were so low in calories. Still, years after I began to follow my fullness program, I was a victim of conditioning. As I ate rich-tasting foods all day long, I associated the rich tastes with immediate weight gain, and I had to run to the scale to reassure myself that my conditioning was wrong and my intellect was right and that I was as slender as ever.

# CHAPTER 6

# How We Began

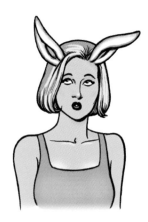

WE HAVE COME SO FAR TOGETHER that I would like to share with you the birth and development of my fullness program. I have told you how I was determined to remain slender, even if I had to live on celery stalks and skim milk. I am not a masochist, so I resented this constant feeling of hunger. Way down deep I also feared that I might fall off the wagon. How long can anyone go without eating some kind of sweet, rich food? I was intrigued by Slim·Fast's promise: "two rich and filling shakes a day and a sensible dinner, and you will be full and slender." But the Slim·Fast product didn't do the trick for me. I decided I should make my own shake to be a part of the fullness plan I was developing.

My friends and I are lucky enough to be women of leisure. In addition, I am lucky enough to have a husband who would back our project financially. We also had the confidence of ignorance. How hard could it be to create a shake and a bar that are rich and filling? We honestly thought that it would take us no more than a year to complete and that the cost would be about $100,000. We were off by 500% on both accounts. It took us more than five years to achieve the US patent for our shake, and the cost ran to more than $500,000.

Rena, Eve and I never divided the work formally, but soon after we started, our natural inclinations led us to take on different responsibilities. I, of course, read all the latest releases on diet and nutrition. I also explored the supermarkets and health-food stores. I know the ingredients and calories by heart. A friend said that it's as if I have my doctorate in nutrition. It was my job to check the ingredients of the diet products on the market. We set up tables of these ingredients and methodically tried one after the other. We also consulted with the top nutritional centers. Both Rutgers and

Cornell have government-sponsored programs to help new food businesses grow and prosper. The nutritionists and technicians at Rutgers were as helpful as could be. It was at Cornell, however, that we established the closest personal relationships. They were with us from the beginning, and five years later, we celebrated the triumph of the patent with a big celebration at Cornell.

Rena took it on herself to establish personal relationships with the technical consultants at companies that provided milk products, chocolate, vitamins, trace minerals, sweeteners, flavorings, and, above all, fibers and gums. When we market our shake, we will do our best to have our manufacturers use the products of the companies whose technicians helped us over the years. Rena also kept meticulous records of all the experimentation that was done, and she finalized the formulations that were necessary for our patent application.

Eve is our baby but is old enough to be our mother. She was always there to organize the correspondence and the bills and the bank records and do countless miscellaneous tasks that Rena and I threw in her lap. Rena and I consider ourselves real workers. Eve is 82, but she outdid both of us in sheer industriousness. We could never have achieved the patent without her.

Cecil, my husband, has been a constant support and constructive critic on both the shake and the book. He supported us from the beginning, and he hosted our weekend celebration at Cornell after we got the patent five years later.

Greg — Dr. Northrop — is Rena's husband. He is a physicist and works on the cutting edge of computer development. We had mountains of detailed studies piled before us. It was Greg who analyzed them and, in 16-column spreadsheets, organized the complex details into crystal-clear solutions.

Our activities were divided into two parts. The first was to make our shake and bar not only delicious but also very filling. We had to bite the bullet and accept the fact that the products we wanted were going to be much more expensive than the other products on the market. There are fibers and gums that can thicken the product, but they are not of the highest grades or quality. To get the mouth-feel and the filling qualities that would last for hours requires a blend of special gums of the very highest quality. These would make the manufacturing cost of our product more than double the cost of the other products on the market. This cost was compounded by the choice of the most expensive chocolate and other flavorings, vitamins and trace minerals and fat fighters, etc. It is our conviction that dieters will be happy to pay more for a delicious bar and shake that fill them up thereby leading to weight loss. The result of all this imagination, effort, and lavish ingredients was a shake and a bar that dazzled the consumer. At Cornell we offered a triple-blind taste test to the faculty and other nutrition authorities. The results fulfilled our highest hopes. The immediate response to our shake and bar was a unanimous rave. The taste and mouth-feel were dimensions away from our competitors' products. Our second test came four hours later. We polled the participants to find out how full they felt after sampling our shake and bar, as compared with their reactions to our competitors' products. Again, there was no contest. Our shake and bar were so incredibly delicious and filling that we won hands-down.

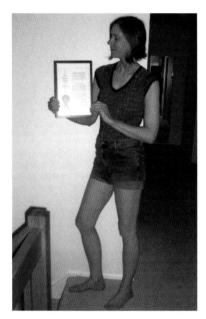

*Celebrating the formal granting of the patent*

When we formulated our bar and shake and achieved our patent, we received offers from major distributors who were eager to put our product on the market. We thought we had achieved our dream, but the fates decreed otherwise. For many decades Atkins was a player in the field of nutrition. His doctrine of weight control by avoiding carbohydrates and living on fat and protein had a core group of followers. This core group kept changing as one follower after another felt that life wasn't worth living without a bite of birthday cake. As time went on, one deprivation diet after another bit the dust. The insidious teaching was that the deprivation diet — and they were all deprivation diets — was successful. The failure was in the sinfully weak dieter who had no character or willpower and so fell off the wagon. The end result was that one famous sure-fire diet after another bit the dust. Atkins grew in power until he became the core of a billion-dollar empire. He seemed unique in that his diet was not based on hunger — his followers could eat all the bacon and eggs and cheese that they desired. He chose to deprive his followers of carbs. This last major deprivation diet ruled the roost. The yellow low-carb label and the triangle red A for Atkins label dominated the supermarket. Thirty-five hundred products labeled themselves "low carb."

The bubble burst as it had to. The insanity of living on fat and protein and the long-term damage to the human organs became evident. Even more damaging was the fact that the dieter began to realize that Atkins was as much a deprivation diet as any other. He allowed you to eat all you wanted to eat but only of a very limited range of foods. The other diets limited the amount of food you could eat. Atkins limited the kind of food you could eat. When the Atkins bubble burst, the whole diet field felt the body blow. The giant Slim·Fast dropped to a shadow of its former self. The stream of diet books and diet product advertising dwindled to a trickle. Nutraceuticals, which are not governed by the FDA, and workout machines are all that are left. In this dis-

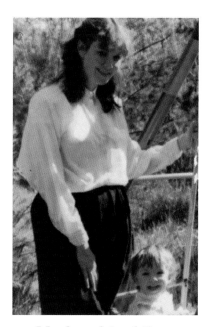

*My dear friend Rena*
*before*

mal atmosphere of disillusionment, the prospects for any new shake or bar, no matter how patented and delicious and filling, were minimal. We had to wait until this disillusionment was over to launch our products.

Rena, Eve, and I met around 1985 and launched our project five years later. Our energies were focused on developing our bar and shake, but we also spread our wings into other areas, mostly related to nutrition. There were over 300 diet books published since 1950. We actually bought and perused at least 20 of them. Many of them showed evidence of hard work and imagination. Some of them actually helped us direct our research. The Cambridge Diet and University Diet and Optifast were shakes that were certainly in the right direction, but they were not filling and many had sugar, which worked against the goal of weight loss. They still were variations of a stalk of celery, plus cottage cheese, plus an eighth of a melon, and skim milk. They did the only thing they could do. They had to cut calories by resorting to gerbil foods — foods without sugar or fat. The result of these 300 diet books and an infinite number of magazine articles was that the obesity indexes climbed alarmingly. It is sad to read about people who tried to heal polio victims with mineral water. It couldn't work, but they had to try something. It's with the same feeling of sadness that we read of all those old diets.

**They were trying their best, but the diets didn't work and couldn't work. They just didn't know then what we know now. The hunger mechanism cannot be resisted. Dieting does not lead to weight loss. The weight everyone loses at the beginning of a diet is not gone. It is put into a bank. After a couple of months the weight comes back, with interest.**

There will be a resurgence of interest in real calorie-cutting products. The threat of obesity is growing, not diminishing. The hunger diets are self-defeating. They are impossible to maintain. Most people just can't live in constant hunger. Even when there is some weight loss, the dismal fact is that the body adjusts to hunger by metabolizing food more efficiently. Given that 3,500 calories equals one pound, if a woman weighing 130 pounds drops 500 calories a day, she should lose a pound a week. The arithmetic is simple. Seven times five is 35. In seven days, losing 500 calories a day, she would have lost 3,500 calories, which comes to a pound of weight. She would lose four pounds a month — which I consider to be the ideal rate of weight loss.

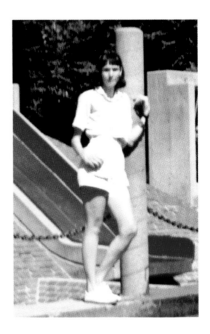

*Rena after*

This premise was logically sound and was unquestioned. It wasn't until fairly recently that physiologists discovered the subtleties of the human metabolism. We are structured to survive even in time of hunger. When there is less food available, our metabolism becomes more efficient so that we can maintain pretty much the same weight while ingesting fewer calories. The tragic result was that the woman who weighed 130 pounds and cut her diet by 500 calories per day would at the end of her dieting weigh pretty close to 130 pounds. Then, when she returned to her pre-diet, 2,500 calories per day — the same calorie level on which she had maintained a weight of 130 pounds — she would now add weight to the tune of one to five pounds. It was a dieter who said sardonically, "If you want to put on weight, go on a diet." Only my fullness program fulfills the need of fullness on low calories.

We are not going to bore you by citing the tons of documentation that indicate sharply that hunger diets are self-defeating and pernicious. Our research for this project turned up one authority after another who blame the hunger diets (and all diets except ours are hunger diets) for being important causes of the obesity epidemic. The yo-yo effect of losing weight for a short period and regaining it with interest in the following period has led our nation's metabolism to put on more weight with fewer calories. The hunger diets have tried to put out the flames of obesity by pouring gasoline onto those flames. The diet industry collects more than $50 billion a year, and the dieters collect ever more fat in their arteries.

Even before physiologists knew about this tragic nuance of our metabolism, a sense of hopelessness pervaded the weight-loss field. Jane Brody, the longtime diet editor of *The New York Times* said that no diet was effective, and Thomas Wadden headed a government study that announced the same conclusion that "there is no known method of achieving permanent weight loss." The globesity indicators were going off the charts. Doctors coined the phrase "syndrome X" to include the prime killers — high blood pressure, diabetes, and heart disease — that are all directly connected with obesity. One doctor I know said, "When experts gather to discuss the future of globesity, they just throw up their hands."

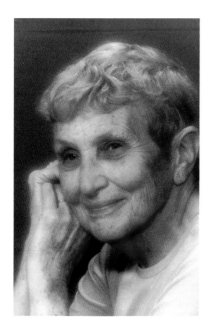

*Eve at 80*

The United Nations announced for the second year that globesity has replaced all other diseases as the single killer threatening humankind. We see graphic evidence of the despair in the cessation of diet advertising. The newspapers and airwaves used to be clogged with ads for diet shakes and diet programs. Now these are gone. All that are left are sporadic ads for pills and workout machines that can be advertised without FDA approval. Even more dramatic is the absence of diet books in the bookstores. The center table on entering a bookstore was classically devoted to the latest diet books. At one time, four of the top 10 *New York Times* best-sellers were diet books. Now there is a pitiful handful of diet books buried in the cooking section. The indicators of obesity are ever more in the red zone. There aren't even books pretending to face this epidemic. It is such good fortune that the wonder foods are increasing in number daily and that the obvious answer to the epidemic of obesity is before us. Science has given us the foods that enable us to eat richly and slim down. We finally have the means of being full on low calories.

# CHAPTER 7

# Tips on Getting Started

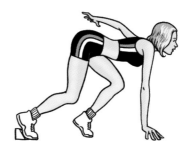

A SUCCESSFUL DIET has three requirements; fun, fun, and fun. This has been the single ingredient missing from other diets. They focus on hunger. They tell you to suffer. My diet is based on emotional and physical fullness, and it works. The experts agree that dieting (hunger) makes the body cling to fat. Repeated dieting results in the yo-yo effect. Hunger makes you lose weight ever more slowly; it makes you regain fat ever more quickly.

My diet is based on the converse of this fact. Just as hunger makes you lose weight ever more slowly, fullness makes you shed weight ever more rapidly. This is proven in the animal world and is the experience of my colleagues and of me.

## I ASSUME THAT:

- You will follow normal nutritional guidelines such as taking a daily multivitamin and checking with your doctor before starting any weight loss program.

- You are an "up" person like me. That you want to consider housework, parking far from the store and avoiding the elevator as fun activities.

- You know that drinking plenty of 0-calorie liquids (black coffee, any tea, diet sodas and water, water, water) is basic to any diet.

- You make a point of varying your foods and drinks and flavors constantly.

- You will keep a tally of your calories as you go through your day. Smoke Enders is a highly successful anti-cigarette program. It demands that the smoker make a note of the number of cigarettes that he lights. The process of writing brings actions to consciousness. You will be delighted when you see the amount of food you have eaten — all within your calorie parameters. At the end of the day, after you've totaled the numbers of calories you have eaten, you might well find that you have fallen short of the total in your plan. If you do have calories left over, you must eat them *today*. In my transition days I would make up the calories in the form of jellybeans or other gold coins. It was delightful to have to eat those extra tidbits. I repeat, at any sign of hunger run, don't walk, to the nearest Gold Coin and return to the state of healing fullness.

- You will use the daily menus as a guide to my "full" way of eating.

- You will have the ego and intelligence to personalize your own eating pattern. Though your calorie total may let you eat 24 fat-free hot dogs or 10 cartons of Egg Beaters for your 1,280 calorie day, you will choose to follow the intelligent guidelines I suggest.

MAKE YOUR OWN RAINBOW OF FOODS. In my transition period I based my day on my ideal weight of 140 pounds. The dietician's rule for weight loss is to take your own goal weight and multiply it by 10. The average person burns 13 calories a day per pound of weight. If you eat fewer calories per day you will reach your ideal weight sooner. Following my program you will be full on 10 calories per pound during this slimming down period. Then you will return, at your own speed, to the normal 13 calories per pound of your ideal weight. The heart of my program is the fun menus that makes you feel full on a minimum of calories.

# CHAPTER 8

# Say Yes to "No-No" Foods

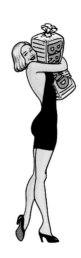

## BREAD

### Recipe 1. Bread and Butter

Everyone loves bread and butter in various forms. Ordinarily these luxurious basics are splurges for the calorie conscious. Bread has always 80 calories an ounce (a slice). Butter is a whopping 100 calories per tablespoon. In olden days bread and butter were indulgences economically. Butter, the fat of the land, was a symbol of wealth. Today the indulgence is not in money but in calories. A couple of slices of regular bread and butter are sinfully caloric.

Switch to my bread and butter and let the magic begin. Science, which has given us so many fattening fast foods, has also given us low-calorie repasts. The slice of bread in whatever form drops in calories from 80 to 40. The sinful butter dwindles from 100 calories per tablespoon to 5 calories. The bread or toast, slathered with butter, drops in calories from a wicked, fattening 180 to a luscious total of 45. Unbelievable — but true.

### Recipe 2. Cinnamon Toast

An universal favorite. This caloric monster would have all the calories of recipe number 1 plus an additional 25 calories for the sugar in its old form. Made with Splenda or other artificial sweetener it is still the miraculous 45 calories (cinnamon has no calories).

### Recipe 3. Ordinary Toast and Jam (or Jelly)

To the 2 slices of toast (160 cal) add 200 calories for 2 tablespoons of butter and 100 calories for 2 tablespoons of jam or jelly, for a wicked total of 460 calories. Our total is 80 cal for the bread, 10 for the butter and 0 cal for the jams or jelly. The total is a slender 90 cal. I repeat that the only difference between the low calories slices and the regular slices is that the low calorie has more fiber and is more healthful. The taste is identical.

## Recipe 4. Peanut Butter and Jelly

The old fattening peanut butter and jelly sandwich is composed of 2 slices of bread (160 cal) 2 tablespoons peanut butter (200 cal) and 1 tablespoon jelly (50 cal). My peanut butter and jelly sandwich is composed of 2 slices of light bread (80 cal), 1 tablespoon Walden Farms peanut spread (0 cal) and 1 tablespoon Walden Farms or other no calorie jelly (0 cal). My total is a luscious 80 calories instead of the standard 410 calories.

## Recipe 5. Waffles

Fattening waffles are 120 calories apiece, a tablespoon of butter is 100 calories, a quarter cup of syrup is 200 calories, for a fattening total of 420 calories per waffle — and who can eat only one? A fat-free waffle is 80, my butter is 5, and my syrup is 0 calories for a total of 85 calories per waffle. THIS IS ONE OF MY PERSONAL STANDARD BREAKFASTS.

## Recipe 6. French Toast

> 1/4 cup skim milk
> 2 Tbs. eggbeater
> 1 drop vanilla extract
> 1 packet Splenda
> Sprinkle of ground cinnamon
> 3 slices light bread

Combine all ingredients except bread in a small bowl. Heat a non-stick skillet and spray lightly with Pam. Dip the bread in the liquid mixture to coat both sides of each piece. Brown the bread in the heated skillet. Serve topped with Promise Ultra fat-free margarine and Walden Farms no calorie syrup for a 160 calorie Festive breakfast feast.

# MAYONNAISE

THERE ARE JOKES about the basic food groups of our day. Among these are the comments that the basic food groups of teenagers are potato chips, pizza and French fries. I am quite serious in suggesting that a basic "food group" should be mayonnaise. It is already a staple of the American diet. No one can eat egg salad, tuna salad or potato salad without mayonnaise. These popular foods become popular because of the mayonnaise in them. The degree of their richness depends on the percentage of mayonnaise they contain. The mother would like to slather mayonnaise onto the salads to make them delicious for the family. She knows, however, that mayonnaise is shamefully caloric — 100 calories per tablespoon. Today's mother is aware of the increase of obesity around her. She is torn by her desire to make the foods as delicious as possible while, at the same time, keeping mayonnaise (calories) to a minimum.

This is an excellent example of the beauty of our new foods. Whatever fat-free mayonnaise might have been when it was first developed, it is now perfected to a point where it tastes even better than its fatty brother. It has the same aroma and taste without the fatty aftertaste and it is only one tenth the calories (10 calories per tablespoon). Old prejudices die hard. Hellman's was the "whole egg" 100 calories per tablespoon choice mayonnaise of the past. The fatty, high calorie product has long been considered the only acceptable mayonnaise to be used by the particular mother. Few of my friends would ever serve food prepared with Kraft fat-free mayonnaise — the one I find most delicious.

A pundit said "I never liked Mark Twain 'till I read him." Some of my friends and relatives don't like the new foods because they won't try them. They have never had a jar of Kraft Fat Free mayonnaise in their pantries. When they visit my home I sometimes have to create white lies. "Of course this is real mayonnaise. Would I serve you anything else?" My visitor eats the mayonnaise happily because there is no way in the world that she could tell it from its fatty twin. The only difference is that her mouth feels cleaner because of the lack of fat in my product. I justify myself for my fib because I am giving her a much more healthful product than the one she thinks she is eating. I long ago gave up thought of convincing the Puritan about the wonder of these new foods. To her they are and will always be "artificial, full of chemicals and absolutely inedible by civilized humans." To have food that is both delicious and low calorie somehow seems sinful to her.

I tried to analyze the Puritan's hostility to the new foods. It is true that some of the

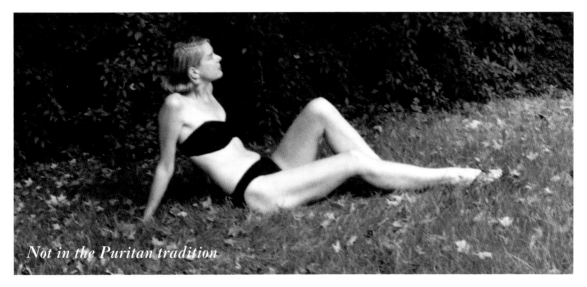

*Not in the Puritan tradition*

new foods were second-rate when they first came on the market. Soldiers in the second war made jokes about the nastiness of their Spam rations. Egg substitutes were sorry products. Butter substitutes were worse. The dairy lobby in Congress fought bitterly against any form of substitute butter. The state of Wisconsin, "the dairy state," passed a law that margarine can be sold in that state only if it is colored black. Vested interests in the old foods work like demons to besmirch the reputation of the new foods. We have discussed the power of the sugar interests in getting cyclamates banned.

The Puritan's tradition has also made it difficult for her to enjoy the new foods. She was trained that if food preparation isn't laborious and painful then the food can be no good. She speaks with contempt about lazy neighbors who destroy their offspring by giving them "dinners out of cans and packages." Long ago Pillsbury put out a cake mix that produced a rich, moist dessert. It didn't sell. They changed the formula so that Puritans had to add eggs to the mix. Then the mix sold. Go figure!

Parallel with the Puritanical objection to the ease of the preparation of these new foods is the prejudice against their price. In tests at the super markets the upper class chooses the most expensive product. The woman who can choose between two identical cans of peas usually chooses the can that costs more. Since it is more expensive it has to be better. This prejudice still dies hard. I gave a talk to a group of women in which I lauded the fat-free hot dog as a staple for the family diet. One woman in the audience said candidly, "but the Oscar Mayer fat-free hot dog cost so much less than the regular hot dogs. I just couldn't serve that kind of food to my family." She made no bones about it. Less expensive meant inferior.

Some people may find it an emotional shock to buy these new foods, which are easily prepared and often less expensive than their caloric twins. If there is any trace of prejudice in you, overcome it. Dare to buy fat-free mayonnaise, your loving Mother would want you to (I feel that Kraft's is the best). Get rid of the old dilemma. Stop choosing between giving your families either healthy foods or delicious foods. With 10 calories per tablespoon you lavish mayo on the family food and still keep the food low calorie. After your plunge into the world of 10-calorie mayo your family will luxuriate in rich egg salad, tuna salad, potato salad, sandwiches of every sort and honor you as being the Chef Extraordinaire. You will be smugly happy giving your family these delicious foods while safeguarding their health.

## BOO'S BACON BITS

THE BEST SPICE for the quiche was bacon bits (*see my quiche recipe on page 93*). This super-low calorie, super low-fat bacon product has come a long, long way from its colorful ancestry. Originally the pig was the wild boar. It was the fiercest and most savage of beasts. Novels of the 19th century tell of the Hapsburg royal hunting parties that were boar hunts. Killing a wild boar was a more difficult feat than killing a lion or tiger. The boar was the totem animal and so was forbidden food for peoples from Jews to Moslems. To people who could eat the animal it was considered a delicacy. Charles Lamb wrote a facetious story about the origin of cooking. He described the ancient days when people ate raw meat. His essay on roast pig was ostensibly a dissertation on the accidental discovery of the benefits of cooked meat. One day a pig farmer suffered a fire in his pigsty. He entered to clean out the dead animals and touched a hot carcass and put his hand to his lips. It was the first time anyone had tasted roast pig. Soon all the neighboring farmers were having fires in their pigsties. This apocryphal story later entered some textbooks as a fact of history. As a literary work the essay is most vivid in its exaltation of roast pigskin, crackle, as one of the special experiences of the human palate.

Pork has had a mixed review nutritionally. In China there is a year called the year of the pig. Certainly there are famous pork dishes in most cultures. Still, the noble savage boar descended to the depths of being a "fat pig." As pigs were bred for lard they became the symbol of obesity. The pig is also that rare animal that soils his own bed. A pigsty is at once the pig's home and his toilet. Add to that the scourge of trichinosis. This is found in many undercooked meats but is most closely identified with pork. Like ecoli, trichinosis is a terrible disease. Once you are afflicted with it you're never the same again.

The pig became the last resort of the poor sharecropper before the Civil War. The cash crop of the South was cotton. Year after year the farmer depleted his soil with his single crop. Finally the cotton plant just wouldn't grow. The last resort of the tenant farmer was to grow corn. This was fed to pigs and the pig became the staple food.

The novel *Mandingo* is a classic about a whole plantation that reached this point. Since they could no longer grow cotton the only cash crop left to them was to grow slaves. They fed the slaves corn, bacon and collard greens. They used selective breeding to establish bloodlines as in racehorses. They had no compunction about mating family members to get the bloodlines they wanted for their cash crop-slaves. This vicious industry was based on the corn-pig cycle.

From this varied background, mostly negative, the pig is stigmatized as a lesser creature than the cow etc. Pork, bacon and lard all have negative overtones. The industry has tried to change the image with an advertising campaign, "pork — the other white meat." The campaign has had little effect.

From this less than stellar background the pig has emerged as one of my favorite food animals. The old fatty bacon has given way to the low calorie, low cholesterol delicious bacon bits. There is no end to uses for this smoky, savory seasoning. Bacon bits are the heart of the piquancy of the low-calorie quiche that I make all the time. They are an important addition to the no-calorie salad dressing. I have used bacon bits as a dressing in itself. I have used bacon bits in seasoning hot vegetables and in casseroles. To those who have any question about the nitrates to be found in bacon bits there is a soy bacon bit that is absolutely acceptable in taste and texture without the nitrates.

I have expanded my use of bacon bits as a smoky, tangy flavoring for dish after dish. So far I have had only positive reactions from my guests. Try your own hand at using this special garnish. I think you will be pleasantly surprised at its versatility. The once despised pig has come into his own.

# CHAPTER 9

# Lordly Shopping in The Land of Plenty

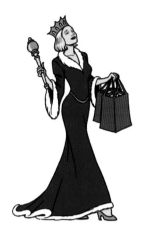

IT IS AN OLD ASSUMPTION that the more food available the more everyone eats and the fatter everyone becomes. There is real logic behind this outlook. The belief was that having good food readily at hand leads one to indulge more freely and to become more obese. I discuss this truism in my lecture at Cornell. What had once seemed obvious turned out to be the reverse of the truth. In spring and summer when the bear was surrounded by plentiful food he evacuated excess food and remained slender. When faced with the lack of food in the winter the bear stored every excess calorie as fat. The seeming logic of keeping the pantry bare actually led to obesity.

Today's psychologists agree that looking on food as an enemy and fearing each meal as another step to obesity results in rapid gluttonous eating and in the very obesity that one dreads. There are new nutrition books written on the French. The French talk about food and dream about food as a natural part of the daily routine. Taking two hours for a leisurely lunch is a matter of course. The French violate the basic rules. Their sauces are calorie rich. The end result of their loving relationship with food is that they suffer far less obesity and far less of the accompanying ailments.

It is time that we emulate the French and establish our own loving relationship with our food. The process is well begun. We no longer have to toil to prepare our daily meals. It seems like ancient history to us that our great-great-grandparents churned milk to make butter and carried the corn to the miller to grind for their bread. Incidentally, the millstones which ground the flour also ground each other. The stone powder in the flour ground down our forefathers' teeth. Yes, these laborious preparations are now in the past. We also have the makings of the world's best relationship with food because we have supermarkets beyond compare. There are still upper class

European ladies who either go or send their maids to the dairy store for milk and cheese and the bakery and the green grocer and the butcher shop and the fish market for their particular products. We could have the best relationship in the world with our food except for the fact that the old prejudices still exist. We are reluctant to be surrounded by lots of delicious food. Having tons of succulent meals around us might result in our overindulgence and obesity. This is the old fashioned fallacy that still cripples us. The acquisition of large amounts of superbly prepared meals has no down side. Its first benefit is that the quantity of good food will lead to slenderness. The bear is at his peak of slenderness in just those seasons when food is most plentiful. That obsolete notion that the empty cupboard leads to slenderness must be reversed. In time of famine, people cram food ravenously and walk around with distended bellies. In the lavish plenty of a three fork French bistro the diner sups graciously and walks away slender and healthy.

The health and the slenderness are the obvious boon of the plentiful larder. There are, however, other benefits. One such benefit is that food shopping becomes a monthly excursion rather than a constant ordeal. Most modern foods have almost unlimited shelf life. Canned food from the American Civil War has been opened and found absolutely fine. Frozen foods last perfectly in your freezer for months. The expiration dates on your cold cuts and cheeses and butter are weeks or months in the future. I do major food shopping only about once a month. Between my major shoppings I casually pick up lettuce, milk and a couple of other perishables. The vestiges of the old pattern of food shopping several times a week are exactly that, vestiges of a long gone era when constant shopping was necessary. Long range shopping is a family bonding time. The variety of delicious food products enables all the family to compare notes on the monthly shopping tour and to make individual tastes and family wide tastes bonding experiences for the family. Shopping as a constant chore is replaced by food shopping as a rewarding family excursion.

When I wrote these chapters the cost of filling our gasoline tank was a few dollars. The price of staples had just begun to soar. By now exorbident prices and living from paycheck to paycheck have become commonplace.

The basic realities have not changed. The indicators of obesity are more on the rise than ever. The need for some kind of weight control is more pressing than ever. Every medical convention, every PTA meeting cries out for some effective program of weight control. Now we have the problem of obesity facing us and the additional problem of poverty. Weight control has always been a very costly process. I have recounted how I tried to follow some of the simple recipes offered by some of the major figures in the field. Their proposals were for individualized programs, usually starting with "an eighth of a melon" and going on to exotic concoctions of 4 ounces of fillet of sole marinated in olive oil and chopped basil. This is hardly the fare of a middle class family after a day at work and at school. In addition to being unmanageable the recipes were wasteful and costly.

One aspect of our way of eating is the incredible thrift involved. The expense of our program is the effort of moving the shoppers arm from the shelf with Kraft 100 calories per tablespoon mayonnaise to the one with Kraft 10 calories per tablespoon mayonnaise; ditto for bread, sour cream, butter, eggs, cheese, frozen dinners, etc. Good begets good. The effective, low-calorie food that is the only real weight control food happens also to be readily available and less expensive. It is the only diet food I know of that does not have the premium cost of all other diets foods.

Long range food shopping is a substantial money saver. With well stocked larder and freezer to begin with the long range shopper focuses on the sale items. The money savings are impressive. Home economists estimate that food costs are cut by over twenty percent when the shopping is optional rather than compulsory.

Long range shopping gets rid of that nagging question of "What shall we have for dinner tonight?" The lines of frozen foods that I have specified are prepared by health conscious, taste conscious, calorie conscious expert chefs. They come in individual size or family portions. Dinner is no longer a matter of compromise; it is a matter of individual and family fulfillment. Finally, long range shopping wipes out the fear of the unexpected. "Company is coming" is a signal for delight rather than for panic.

Long range shopping is healthful, economic, a source of family unity, etc.etc., but it is also the exception rather than the norm. Cultural lag can take a heavy toll. The first refrigerators were regarded with suspicion as "containing poison gas." Canned and frozen foods are still suspect by many "good housewives." I, myself, sometimes look longingly to the fresh vegetable section of the supermarket. After all my years in the field of nutrition the old prejudices still haven't died completely. I sometimes forget that canned and frozen foods are processed immediately after being picked in the field. I believe that canned foods have more vitamins and are fresher that the vegetables the farmer brings home to his wife that evening. Similarly, the old prejudices make me look to the fresh fish section. It takes little imagination to know the obvious truth that the fish were frozen immediately after being caught at sea. The "fresh fish" were caught days ago, packed in ice and, shipped to the fish store. The frozen fish were kept in perfect state moments after being caught. The frozen fish are superior in every way to the "fresh." Since traces of the old fashioned outlook still linger in my mind, and I am a devotee of nutrition, I understand how hard it may be for you to break into the pattern of long range food shopping. It is however the way to go. Long range food shopping has no down side. Try to overcome your old prejudices and join the 21st century.

Melding your personal fullness program into the family food program can be a delightful exercise. Be selfish. Make your own dietary requirement the first priority. Your family will be the beneficiary of your new slenderness. Start with the nutrition for which our country is most famous. Our country leads the world in bad, fatty hamburgers and pizza. We are also the creators of delicious lines of basics which can easily turn simple proteins into my program's kind of meals — tasty, filling and low-calorie.

There are at least a dozen meal starters like Hamburger Helper by Betty Crocker. They are popular, but not nearly as popular as they should be. We're again faced with grandma's prejudice that easy, delicious foods are products of the devil. These starter foods provide sauces, spices, vegetables etc. that make up truly gourmet dinners. All the master chef has to do is to add either hamburger or tuna fish or chicken or other staple proteins to complete the chef d'oeuvre — the masterpiece.

Among the other boons of this kind of dinner is the calorie count. The package specifies the calories and also the calories of the pound of meat or fish or other protein to be added. When the dish is served, your job is to lop off the caloric portion that you choose for your program. The rest goes to the peasants around the table, your mate and children. You and they will revel in your gourmet creation.

With all these family dishes before you the great fun is to let your imagination run wild among the scores of foods that fit my criteria. I use chicken in various forms many times a month. I use hamburger in its various forms several times a month. I use fish occasionally; I should feature fish more often. I've found dozens of meal-in-a-bag type dinners that are superb. This kind of planning causes an emotional reversal. Instead of the daily ordeal of trying to answer that nagging question of, "What are we having for dinner tonight?" I now am a queen who can choose among the many delicacies at hand.

# Festive Desserts!

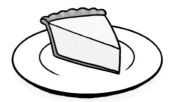

## CHEESECAKE

A classic of Broadway theatre is "Guys and Dolls." Theatre groups across the country have made Nathan Detroit and Nicely Nicely Johnson part of American folklore. The play evolves in a setting of Lindy's Deli in the heart of the Broadway theatre district. There the characters read the racing forms and plan the next floating crap game while eating Lindy's famous cheesecake. Many tourists make Lindy's a part of their visit to partake of the legendary cheesecake.

Lindy's cheesecake is famous but also very caloric. Witness the avoirdupois of the Damon Runyan characters. Now modern technology gives us the glory of Lindy's New York Cheesecake without the penalty of the accompanying rolls of fat. Lindy's New York Cheesecake is made up principally of 2 and a half pounds of cream cheese (4,000 calories), 2 cups of sugar (1548 calories), heavy whipping cream (400 calories), egg yolks (180 calories), whole eggs (400 calories), flour (475 calories), butter (813 calories) etc. For details of this classic recipe see the *New York Cookbook* by Molly O'Neill.

My "Guys and Dolls" are slim, trim and gorgeous. Instead of the Lindy's 868 calories a serving, my cheesecake is just as dense, rich and sinfully delicious as theirs is, and weighs in at less than 300 calories a serving. Here's how the magic is done.

Boo's Cheesecake

    3 packages (8oz. each) Philadelphia fat-free cream cheese, softened

1 cup bulk Splenda (the one in the box — not the new bulk Splenda
made with added sugar)
1/2 cup Breakstone fat free sour cream
2 Tbs. cornstarch
1/2 cup Egg Beaters
2 tsp. vanilla extract
4 graham cracker squares, crumbled

Blend all ingredients except graham crackers. Line bottom of a 9-inch spring-form pan with waxed paper. Spray the sides with Pam. Make sure that the ingredients are blended into a smooth consistency then pour mixture into pan. Bake in 325-degree oven 43 minutes, or just until soft set in center. Remove from oven and run a knife along outside of cheesecake. Let cool on rack to room temperature. Top with crumbled graham crackers. You will top Marie Antoinette with "Let them eat cheesecake." 1/8 cake serving is only 138 calories.

## BOO'S BROWNIES

There is nothing new under the sun. None of the ingredients or processes that I use is original to me: they have all been used before. The unique thing about my Fullness Program is my approach.

Non-sugar recipes are largely to be found in diabetic cookbooks. Low-fat diets are usually used therapeutically. They are used defensively and apologetically. If you are sick you can use a sugar substitute. If you are fat you can use low-fat products. A friend once compared my approach to diet with a woman's approach to wigs. In our country the wig was used therapeutically and apologetically. If a woman lost her hair because of chemo or other processes she could wear a wig. If her hair is thinning she can wear a wig. The European fashion plate wears her wig proudly. She can change her hairstyle and her appearance in a moment with little effort and with marvelous results in her beauty. The European and the American are both women. The wigs are both wigs. The difference is in the mindset. It is the old question of whether the cup is half empty or half full.

The diabetes cookbook describes the use of sugar-free chocolate pudding apologetically. I find sugar-free chocolate pudding identical in taste to the sugary product when prepared properly. I use this marvelous product as a hot fudge topping and as a pudding unto itself. Today I am using it as the basis for the most sinful of desserts — the walnut fudge brownie covered with whipped cream.

Start with the dream. Imagine a lusciously rich chocolate brownie with walnuts and gobs and gobs of whipped cream topping. This devilish temptation is a horrible 440 calories. "A moment on your lips, forever on your hips."

Now let us hear the blare of trumpets and the beating of drums for the triumphant march. Imagine that same brownie, absolutely delicious, even healthier than the fatty one, but only 125 calories. Here is how to create the magic.

Into a one quart Corning dish put one cup water and one four serving package Jell-O Cook & Serve Sugar-free Chocolate pudding and one tablespoon flour and one packet of Splenda. Add 1 ounce of chopped walnuts and stir. Microwave on high for 2 to 4 minutes. Allow cooling. Now get ready to swoon. On top of this brownie you will squirt four tablespoons of Reddi-wip topping on each quarter.

I don't want to ruin this decadent dessert for you but I have to confess to you that each portion of the brownie has a gram and a half of fiber. The darn brownie is not only sinfully delicious but it is also healthful. Don't leave this goody to the sickly and the diabetic. Enjoy triumphantly.

Boo's Brownies

> One 1.3 oz. Package Cook & Serve sugar free Jell-O chocolate pudding
> 1 Tbs. flour
> 1 cup water
> 1 packet Splenda
> 1 oz. chopped walnuts
> Reddi-wip topping

In a 1 quart microwavable Corning or other dish wisk the pudding powder, flour and the water. Stir in walnuts.

Microwave uncovered on high for 2 to 4 minutes. On your first round watch carefully because microwaves differ in power. After your first batch you'll know the time needed to make the mixture set. Allow to cool. Divide into quarters. Top each serving with four tablespoons Reddi-wip topping. Enjoy.

**MORE RECIPE IDEAS:**

## Chemistry Chocolate Cake

| | |
|---|---:|
| 1 cup cake flour | 360 cal |
| 3 Tbs. bulk Sugar Twin | 15 cal |
| 3 Tbs. Hershey's cocoa | 30 cal |
| 1 1/4 tsp. baking soda | |
| 1 cup water | |
| 1 Tbs. white vinegar | |
| 2 tsp. vanilla extract | 10 cal |

Put all ingredients together in a 9-inch cake pan. Stir with a spoon until blended. Bake at 350 degrees for 25 minutes. 415 calories for entire cake.
May be baked in non-stick muffin pan. 53 calories for each of 8 servings.

## Orange Dream

| | |
|---|---:|
| 2 cups Stewarts Diet orange 'n cream soda (no calories), or 2 cups Crystal Light Classic Orange (10 calories), or 2 cups Sugar Free Tang (10 calories) | |
| 4 tsp. Deb-El Just Whites powdered egg whites | 24 cal |
| 3/4 tsp. Vanilla extract | 5 cal |
| 1/4 cup bulk Splenda | |
| 1 heaping cup ice | |

Combine all ingredients in a blender and blend on high for one minute. 35 calories made with orange soda, 45 calories made with Crystal Light or Tang.

## Hot Blueberry Dessert

| | |
|---|---:|
| 6–8 packets Splenda | 0 cal |
| 1 bag (2 cups) frozen blueberries | 200 cal |
| 1 1/2 tsp. lemon juice | 2 cal |
| 1/2 Tbs. vanilla extract | 15 cal |
| 1/2 Tbs. almond extract | 15 cal |

| | |
|---|---|
| 1/2 tsp. cinnamon | 3 cal |
| 1/2 Tbs. cornstarch dissolved in 3/4 cup cold water | 22 cal |

Dissolve cornstarch, Combine all ingredients and stir over low heat until thick. Allow to cool and serve. Total recipe is 257 calories.

## Easy Pumpkin Muffins

| | |
|---|---|
| 1 Box Duncan Hines Spice Cake mix | 180 cal for 1/12 of mix |
| 15 oz. can Libby's 100% pure pumpkin | 40 calories per 1/2 cup |
| 1 cup water | |
| 1 tsp. pumpkin pie spice | |
| 8 packets Splenda, or 1/2 - 3/4 cup bulk Splenda, according to taste | |

Combine all ingredients in a large mixing bowl. Stir until blended. Pour into non-stick muffin pans sprayed lightly with cooking spray. Bake according to package directions, 25 to 35 minutes. Makes 12 muffins at 200 calories each. I eat several of these muffins every week.

## Festive Jell-O Whip

| | |
|---|---|
| 1 – 4-serving package sugar free Jell-O (Any flavor, lemon is nice) | 40 cal |
| 1 cup boiling water | 0 cal |
| Diet Ginger ale, or other flavor diet soda compatible with the flavor of Jell-O you use. | 0 cal |

Prepare Jell-O by the "quick set" method on package by dissolving in hot water then adding ice. When the Jell-O has begun to set but isn't yet firm put it in a blender. Add 12 ounces diet soda and blend. You may need to experiment with this one. Vary the set time of the Jell-O and the amount of soda until your Jell-O whip becomes a soft "cloud." 40 calories for entire blender of whipped Jell-O.

*My Favorite Festive Day*

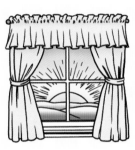

## BREAKFAST

The special Sunday breakfasts of Eggs Benedict or pancakes and sausage are my everyday norm. Easiest, and really my favorite, is the Festive breakfast I describe on the following page. It consists of three slices Wonder Light bread, toasted, three table-spoons of Promise fat-free margarine, Splenda, Turkey Sausage, and unlimited Walden Farms (or other brand) no-calorie pancake syrup.

You must understand that to me this breakfast tastes fatty and is super-filling. Shortly after I began my Fullness Program, focusing on low-fat or no-fat foods, my whole perspective on fat changed. Like most Americans, I grew up on a diet in which fat was a supreme treat. Prime rib, grade-A steak (the grade of beef is based simply on the amount of fat, the more fat the higher the grade), lamb chops, etc., were the treats at mealtimes. Non-fat foods were ho-hum; only fatty foods were the treats.

At times this was carried to excess. An aunt of mine wanted to prepare a treat for her new fiancé. He once expressed his taste for roast pig. The preparation was a comedy of errors. My poor aunt didn't think to measure the size of her oven. She bought the suckling pig just before the holiday and could not exchange it. It just didn't fit. She ended up by cutting it into two halves, and then she tried to serve them together. The point is that we could eat only a couple mouthfuls of the delicious skin, the crackle. The suckling skin was pure fat. After all the buildup we could enjoy only a couple of minutes of this *piece de resistance*. A few mouthfuls of this pure fat, and we were sated. In the laboratory, mice fed on fat ignored other foods. Fat is completely addictive. The converse is also true. Once I adjusted to a diet of protein and carbohydrates with far less than 30 percent fat, I lost my old craving for fat.

Sausage links used to be one of my favorites at family breakfasts. After I became accustomed to my low-fat diet my palate changed. On a visit home I was served my old time favorite and I bit into what used to be my treat. I simply couldn't swallow the fatty meat. My whole metabolism had changed to a point where I had to spit my mouthful of fat sausage into my napkin. Aside from feeling infinitely healthier without the fat I was able to enjoy food and life more than ever before. Eating became dining. Swallowing fat means swallowing nine calories a gram. Ingesting proteins and carbohydrates involves less than half that number of calories per gram. It takes more than twice as long to dine on my present diet than on the one on which I was raised.

Nutritional studies of old cultures are indicative of the benefits of low-fat diets. The ancient Greeks were very long lived. They ate cereal and olives and cheese and some fish. Meat, especially fatty meat, was rare. The bulk of their diet was cereal, cereal, cereal three times a day. In our day we know that the Asian was always lean and slender until the fatty foods hit even Asia.

My breakfast is the simple example of the low-calorie, tasty, filling, readily available foods that can be assembled into a feast. In place of the standard fatty 750 calorie breakfast of bacon, eggs and hash browns you will have enjoyed a low-fat feast for 170 calories.

## Breakfast Recipe

| | |
|---|---|
| 3 slices Wonder Light bread, toasted | 120 cal |
| 3 tablespoons Promise Ultra Fat free Margarine | 15 cal |
| Splenda | 0 cal |
| Unlimited 0 calorie pancake syrup | 0 cal |
| 1 Banquet Turkey sausage | 35 cal |

Microwave sausage. Toast bread. Spread margarine on bread. Pour pancake syrup over everything and sprinkle splenda on top.

*This is my personal breakfast at least 4 mornings a week.*

## LUNCH

I am Spartan in my lunch menus. I am usually pressed for time and eating a Festive lunch can make me sleepy by early afternoon. I often opt to make my lunch from a number of sandwich choices such as: peanut butter and jelly, cucumber and cream cheese, bologna on Weight Watcher's rye (with lettuce or cream cheese) or tuna (*See menu choices on page 42*).

When I do have the time for a Festive lunch I usually indulge in the wonder food pasta called Shirataki described in the section called "Use Your Noodle" on page 111. I dress it with either House of Tsang Classic Stir Fry sauce at 25 calories per tablespoon for a delicious lo mein or with low calorie Healthy Choice or Ragú Light if I'm in the mood for spaghetti. This enormous lunch comes to about 150 calories. It is a luxury to eat a giant bowl of noodles, which, unlike fattening pasta, is both slimming and nourishing you with tons of fiber.

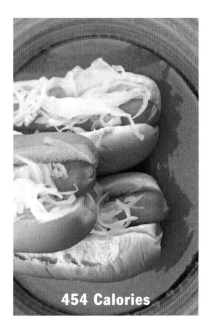

**454 Calories**

## DINNER

**Boo's Hot Dog Dinner:** Nathan's Hot Dog stand offered a special of 3 of their hot dogs for 3 dollars and 33

*Simple, filling hot dog dinner*

cents. Grandma told us that hot dogs were made up of meat from pig's ears and cow's lips and dead mice. During the muckraking period, when big industry was exposed, the meat packers were targeted for what they put into hot dogs. The list is nauseating. It included waste, dead rodents and human fingers. Only a negligent mother would serve her abused children such awful food for their dinner. The word hot dog became anathema to discriminating mothers from 1900 on. This myth still lingers. The truth, though, is that today's hot dog has nothing to do with the awful hot dog of the past. It is made to the same standards as fillet mignon and rack of lamb. Today's hot dog is a perfect meat seasoned to the specification of its brand.

Today's regular, fatty hot dog is good but is ridiculously caloric. This hot dog at one time was a standard snack or meal. It rivaled the hamburger as the American staple. Starting in the '60s, pizza gained ascendancy as the American fast food. Now the trend is turning back to the hot dog and hamburger.

The offer of three full sized hot dogs accompanied with buns, sauerkraut, relish, mustard, etc. for 1 dollar 11 cents apiece is a good food purchase. Don't worry about Nathan's however. They may not make much on the hot dog but they know the high percentage of customers who will also want fries and Cokes. The fries cost them under 15 cents and sell for about a dollar and a half. The Cokes sell for a dollar or more but they cost less than the paper cup in which they are served. Once they get you to buy the hot dog they will come out very well on the whole meal.

My objection is not to the impurity of their food or to the cost. My objection is to the terrible, unnecessary caloric content of the meal. Their hot dog and bun are a total of 310 calories. If one ate the special offer of 3 for 333, the hot dogs would total almost 1,000 calories. This is in addition to the fries, Coke and so on. This is obesity in the making.

A mother following my fullness plan will serve her children the same three hot dogs with all the trimmings. The hot dogs will not be fatty beef; they will be spiced turkey or chicken meat. Each hot dog will be 40 calories; each bun will be 80. The total of the three will be well under 500 calories.

The meal will be accompanied, of course, with diet drinks. The lean hot dog plus the low calorie bun plus lots of sauerkraut will result in a nourishing, satisfying dinner with fiber, protein and carbohydrates. Instead of fearing the old bugaboo of feeding your child hotdogs, know that you are feeding him pure chicken or turkey freer of fat than filet mignon.

Boo's Hot Dog Dinner

| | |
|---|---|
| 3 Oscar Mayer Fat-free hot dogs | 120 cal |
| 3 Wonder Light hot dog buns | 240 cal |
| 14 oz. Can sauerkraut | 74 cal |
| Ketchup, relish, mustard to taste | approx. 20 cal |

Broil, fry in Pam, or microwave hot dogs. Warm buns in microwave or toaster
Drain sauerkraut. Assemble and go to Elizabeth Arden's Red Door for a massage and bubble bath to recover from the ordeal of making this elaborate dinner.

# Festive Meals for the Family

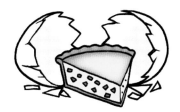

## THE QUICHE OF LIFE

Egg producers are trying to make a comeback. The egg was so maligned during the cholesterol scare that consumption plummeted. Since the egg yolk is full of cholesterol and since cholesterol clogs arteries, eating an egg was equated with eating poison. As late as ten years ago, members of my family would not touch an egg.

Egg producers ran an intensive campaign about the "incredible edible egg." Even more important, medical authorities separated cholesterol in food from cholesterol in the human body. The cholesterol in food goes through the digestive system and does not go directly into the bloodstream. The cholesterol in the bloodstream is manufactured by ones own body and has little relationship to the cholesterol one ingests. Slowly the egg is coming back into favor as an American staple. We are still not back to the point that ham and eggs or bacon and eggs are the standard breakfast of the American family. We may never get back to that point. The egg however is now solidly back as a part of our diet.

My objection to the egg is that it is highly and unnecessarily caloric. A medium sized egg is 70 calories. Most of the calories are in the yolk. Attempts have been made to develop less caloric eggs. In the Second World War the military fed the troops powdered eggs. They were practically inedible. One enterprising mess cook put pieces of eggshell into the mix to fool the troops into thinking that there were fresh eggs involved. The trick didn't work.

Thirty some years ago, Egg Beaters hit the market. They weren't very good. Slowly Fleischmann's and other companies kept improving the product. Now the composition is still ninety-nine percent egg white, super low calorie protein, the annatto coloring and the subtle flavor improvements have taken this non-fat, non-cholesterol, almost purely protein product and enhanced it to the point that, with bacon bits or other flavoring, it is delicious in omelet or other form. The cheese version and garden vegetable version of Egg Beaters are very slightly more caloric but they, also, are excellent.

The special value of my Festive quiche formula is that most adults and almost all children are less than passionate about vegetables. There are many ways of doctoring vegetables. None is as effective, I believe, as my version of the quiche. I propose the quiche, loaded with fat-free cheese and flavored with bacon bits, as my secret weapon in making spinach, zucchini etc. a taste treat for adults and, especially, for children.

The word quiche is a corruption of the German kuchen or cake. Alsace Lorraine is a district that has passed back and forth between Germany and France for centuries. The Germans called it Lothringa; the French called it Lorraine. The popular dish in that area was an egg custard laced with bacon or ham, hence the name Quiche Lorraine. It was imported to our country in the '50s. Since it had no real meat it produced the adage "Real men don't eat quiche." It was the fashionable luncheon food for the garden club crowd. Now, in various forms, it has become an upper class form of pizza.

The Spanish had long eaten cold scrambled eggs (with various inclusions) as a picnic favorite. Huevos Rancheros made it only to the Tex-Mex area of the United States. The cold crustless quiche is an appetizer at posh restaurants like Cipriani's. My proposal is much humbler and more mundane. I have used the Quiche Lorraine mix as, in effect, a sauce or carrier for the much-despised vegetable. Spinach, broccoli, asparagus, bell peppers, onions, mushrooms all go down much easier in a medium of quiche. There is no easier, healthier single dish, luncheon or dinner, than egg batter spiced with bacon bits etc. stuffed full of the healthiest vegetables possible. The pickiest child may well eat his vegetables gladly when they are ensconced in well-seasoned cheese and egg batter. The mother is ecstatic because she is serving her child a fantasy meal of pure protein and fibrous vegetables. The Egg Beaters total is 60 calories for half a cup as compared with 140 calories for nature's inferior product (for 2 "eggs"). Last night I had a truly Festive repast of Egg Beaters, cheese, bacon and spinach for 380 calories, half of the following recipe.

## Quiche of Life

| | |
|---|---:|
| 1 – 8 oz. carton Egg Beaters: | 120 cal |
| 1 – 8 oz. package Kraft Fat-Free shredded cheddar cheese: | 360 cal |
| 1 – 3 oz. jar Hormel 50% less fat real bacon bits: | 200 cal |
| 1 – 9 oz. package frozen spinach, thawed and drained: | 80 cal |

Southwest Version *substitute spinach with:*

| | |
|---|---:|
| 1 – 3oz. jar Hormel 50% less fat real bacon bits: | 200 cal |
| 1 – 4oz. can Ortega Diced Green Chiles: | 30 cal |

Spray a 13 x 9 inch cake pan with All Natural Butter Flavor Pam. Spoon Chiles into 8 mounds in pan. Sprinkle cheese evenly over pan. Spoon bacon bits in 8 mounds into pan and smooth carefully. Tear spinach apart and make 8 mounds around the pan. Smooth. Pour Egg Beaters slowly and carefully over the whole things. Bake, covered, at 350 for 25 minutes. Uncover and bake another 10 minutes.
For appetizer portions cut into 8ths and serve warm.
Dinner could be 1/3 to 1/4 the whole recipe!

**MORE RECIPE IDEAS:**

## Egg Foo Yung

| | |
|---|---:|
| 1/4 cup chopped onion: | 17 cal |
| 14 oz. can bean sprouts: | 53 cal |
| 2 oz. Jennie-O turkey ham diced: | 80 cal |
| 2 cups Egg Beaters: | 240 cal |
| 1/2 Tbs. light soy sauce: | 7 cal |
| 1/2 Tbs. House of Tsang Classic Stir Fry sauce: | 13 cal |
| 1/2 cup fat-free chicken broth: | 15 cal |
| 1 tsp. cornstarch: | 18 cal |
| 1/2 tsp. oil (from spray) for pan: | 20 cal |
| 1 – 1 second spray of oil for each of four servings of Egg Beaters (7 calories each) | |

Sauté vegetables and meat in a non-stick frying pan sprayed with 1/2 teaspoon oil, add stir fry sauce. In a saucepan mix chicken broth and soy sauce, heat on high. In a small bowl mix corn starch and a small amount of cold water, add to sauce and stir over heat until thickened. Pour 1/2 cup Egg Beaters into a non-stick frying pan sprayed with oil. Cook eggbeater until it begins to set and add 1/4 of the meat and beansprout mixture. Fold edges to center making a 4 inch circle. Turn over and brown lightly. Transfer to a plate and pour 1/4 of the sauce over omelet and serve.

Serves four — 470 calories total

117.5 calories for each of four servings.

## Italian Style Chicken Cutlets

| | |
|---|---|
| 1 package Perdue Low Fat Breaded Chicken Breast Cutlets Italian Style | 160 cal each piece |
| 4 one-pound bags frozen sliced zucchini | 100 cal per pound |
| 2 cups Healthy Choice Traditional Pasta Sauce, or Ragú Light Pasta Sauce | 60 cal per 1/2 cup |
| 4 Tbs. fat-free grated Parmesan | 10 cal per Tbs. |

Warm the chicken cutlets in the oven as directed on the package. While the chicken is becoming crisp cook each bag of zucchini separately in the microwave, drain and place on dinner plate. Top each plate of zucchini with 1/2 cup pasta sauce and warm in the microwave a few seconds. Crown each plate with a crisp chicken cutlet and a tablespoon of grated cheese. Each super-filling serving is only 330 calories.

## Breaded Fish Fillets

| | |
|---|---|
| 2 packages Gorton's Parmesan Crunchy Breaded Fish Fillets | 250 cal for 2 fillets |
| (Other flavors of Gorton's fillets also available for same calories) | |
| 4 mini ears Green Giant frozen corn on the cob (extra sweet) | 60 cal ea. |
| 2 one-pound bags frozen broccoli | 125 cal per bag |
| 4 Tbs. Kraft fat-free mayonnaise | 10 cal per Tbs. |
| 4 tsp. B & G sugar free pickle relish | 5 cal per tsp. |
| 4 servings Pam cooking spray | |
| 4 Tbs. Promise Ultra Fat Free margarine | 20 cal |

Prepare fish fillets, corn and broccoli according to package directions. Combine fat-free mayo and relish to make tartar sauce. Assemble 4 Festive dinners each consisting of 2 fillets topped with 1 tablespoon tartar sauce, 1 ear of corn sprayed with Pam and 1/2 lb. Broccoli topped with one tablespoons fat-free margarine. 420 calories for each Festive dinner.

## Polish Sausages

| | |
|---|---|
| 1 package Hillshire Farms Turkey Polish Kielbasa | 2 oz. serving 90 cal |
| 1 package light hot dog buns | 80 cal each |
| 2 bags frozen pepper and onion strips | 125 cal per bag |
| 1/2 cup Breakstone's fat-free sour cream *(optional)* | 15 cal per Tbs. |

Cook peppers and onions in microwave. Heat kielbasa and cut into 2 oz. portions, then cut portions in half lengthwise. Toast 8 buns. Fill each bun with a slice of kielbasa. Assemble each 330 calorie Festive dinner using two sandwiches and 1/4 of the sausage and peppers garnished with one tablespoon fat-free sour cream. Delicious.

## Tamales

| | |
|---|---|
| 2 cans Hormel Hot 'N Spicy Beef Tamales in Chili sauce | 3 tamales for 210 cal |
| 4 oz. Healthy Choice 94% reduced fat shredded cheddar | 40 cal per oz. |
| 12 cups lettuce, shredded | 10 cal per cup |
| 8 tablespoons fat-free sour cream | 15 cal per Tbs. |

Heat tamales in microwave. Place 3 cups shredded lettuce on each of 4 plates. Sprinkle one ounce cheddar over each bed of lettuce. Place 3 tamales on each bed, topped with two tablespoons fat-free sour cream. 310 calories per Festive dinner.

## Corned Beef Hash

| | |
|---|---|
| 1 can Mary Kitchen 50% reduced fat corned beef hash | 290 cal can |
| 1 – 16oz. carton Egg Beaters | 1/2 cup per serving, 60 cal |
| 1 pound frozen green beans | 1/4 lb for 40 cal |
| 4 Ore-Ida Toaster Hash Browns | 110 cal per patty |

Walden Farms Calorie Free Creamy Bacon salad dressing or Dip

Heat the hash in a non-stick skillet. Scramble the Egg Beaters, toast the hash browns and cook the green beans in the microwave. Assemble 4 Festive dinners using 1/2 cup hash, 1/4 of the green beans topped with dressing, 1/4 of the scrambled Egg Beaters and 1 hash brown patty. Each dinner — 350 cal.

## Stuffed Potatoes

| | |
|---|---|
| 4 potatoes each weighing 5 1/2 oz. raw | 120 cal each |
| 8 tablespoons Promise Ultra Fat-free margarine | 5 cal each |
| 2 – 6 oz. cans Bumble Bee tuna in water | 70 cal for 3 oz. |
| 1 – 1 lb. bag frozen broccoli | 1/4 pound 40 calories |
| 4 slices Smart Beat fat-free sharp cheddar cheese | 25 cal each |
| or 8 tablespoons Breakstone fat-free sour cream | 15 cal per Tbs. |

Bake the potatoes or cook in the microwave, as you prefer. Cook broccoli in microwave and divide into 4 portions. Cut each baked potato in half. Mash 3 ounces of tuna and 2 tablespoons margarine into each potato. Top with one portion of broccoli and one slice of cheese and warm briefly in microwave, or warm without the cheese and then top with two tablespoons sour cream. 270 cal for each Festive dinner.

## "Lean Cuisine" Dinner

| | |
|---|---|
| 4 packages Lean Cuisine Santa Fe Style Rice and Beans | 290 cal each |
| 4 – 10 oz. packages chopped broccoli | 105 cal per package |

Cook broccoli in microwave. Heat Lean Cuisine entrees according to package. Assemble each Festive meal by making a bed of one package of broccoli topped with one package of rice and beans. Makes a very satisfying 405 calorie meatless Festive meal. (Look for other frozen low calorie, individual serving entrees and invent your own Festive dinners. An entrée can have up to 350 calories per serving and be combined with up to 100 calories of your favorite vegetable. Get the family in on the adventure. Variety is essential.)

## Festive Chili

| | |
|---|---|
| 2 – 15oz.cans Hormel Turkey or Vegetarian 99% Fat Free Chili | 203 cal per cup |
| 16 cups lettuce, shredded | 10 cal per cup |
| 4 oz. Healthy Choice Fat-Free shredded cheddar | 40 cal per oz. |

Heat the chili. Place 4 cups lettuce on each of four plates. Top each with one cup chili and one ounce cheese. 283 calories for each Festive dinner.

## Tacos

| | |
|---|---|
| 8 oz. roasted skinless chicken breast meat, cubed; | 320 cal |
| or 2 cups Old El Paso fat-free refried beans, warmed | 360 cal |
| 8 Old El Paso ready to serve White Corn Taco Shells | 50 cal each |
| 4 oz. Healthy Choice Fat-Free shredded cheddar | 40 cal per oz. |
| Any brand salsa | 10 cal for 2 Tbs. |
| Breakstone Fat-free sour cream | 15 cal per Tbs. |
| 8 cups lettuce, shredded | 10 cal per cup |

For each dinner assemble two tacos using 2 taco shells, 2 cups lettuce, divided, either 2 ounces of chicken or 1/2 cup refried beans (heat and divide into 1/4 cup for each taco). Top each taco with 1/2 ounce cheddar plus one tablespoon sour cream and one tablespoon salsa. Festive Chicken Taco dinner comes to 153 calories, Festive Bean Taco dinner comes to 163 calories. Serves 4 guests, 2 tacos each! Enjoy.

## Broiled Flounder

| | |
|---|---|
| 4 Individually frozen flounder fillets (Wholey, or other brand) | 130 cal per fillet |
| Pam spray | |
| 4 Ore Ida Toaster Hash Brown Patties | 110 cal |
| **or:** 4 Birdseye frozen mini ears of corn | 80 cal each |
| 3 – 10 oz. Birdseye Green Beans with Almonds | 50 cal per 3 oz. serving |
| (use two servings per Festive dinner) | |

Spray fillets with Pam and bake or broil according to package. Cook the green beans in the microwave and add almonds according to directions. Toast the hash browns, or steam corn according to directions. Assemble each Festive meal with one flounder fillet, 2 servings of green beans with almonds and one toaster hash brown patty or one ear of corn. Each Festive dinner comes to a very filling 330–400 calories.

## Chicken Nuggets

| | |
|---|---|
| 1 – 18-piece package Perdue fun shape chicken nuggets | 190 cal for 4 nuggets |
| 1 package Ore Ida Toaster Hash Browns | 110 cal per patty |
| 2 – 1 lb. bags frozen broccoli | 125 cal per pound |
| 1 jar Heinz Fat Free Chicken gravy | 20 cal per 1/2 cup |

Heat nuggets according to package. Cook broccoli in microwave and divide into 4 portions. Toast hash brown patties in toaster. Assemble each Festive dinner with 1 (1/2 pound) portion of broccoli, topped with 1/2 cup gravy, 4 nuggets and one hash brown patty. 385 calories per Festive dinner.

## Green Giant Pasta Alfredo

| | |
|---|---|
| 2 packages Green Giant frozen Pasta Accents Alfredo | 210 cal for 2 cups |
| 2 – 1 lb. bags frozen broccoli | 65 cal per 1/2 pound |

Cook Pasta Accents Alfredo according to directions. Steam frozen broccoli in microwave. Assemble each portion using 1/4 of the broccoli topped with 2 cups of the Pasta Accents. 275 calories per Festive dinner.

## Banquet Family Entrée Chicken and Noodles

| | |
|---|---|
| 1 package Banquet Family Entrée Chicken and Noodles | 210 cal per 8 oz. serving |
| 2 – 1 lb. bags frozen cut green beans | 165 calories per pound |

Prepare Banquet Entrée according to directions. Steam green beans in microwave and divide into 4 portions. Assemble each portion using 1/2 lb. of green beans and one (8oz.) serving of chicken and noodles. 300 calories per portion.

**There are a number of easily prepared meals in boxes, offered on the grocery store shelves, which lend themselves to our festive way of life. For Example:**

### Betty Crocker Complete Meals: Homestyle Chicken and Dumplings

| | |
|---|---|
| 1 package Betty Crocker Complete Meals Homestyle Chicken and Dumplings | 250 cal for 1/5 box |
| 2 – 1 lb. bags frozen broccoli | 50 to 80 calories per 1/2 pound |
| or: equivalent amount frozen cauliflower, green beans, any vegetable you like | |
| 1 jar Heinz Fat Free Chicken Gravy | 20 cal per 1/4 cup serving |

Prepare Complete Meal according to package. Cook vegetables in microwave. Heat gravy. Assemble each 350 calorie dinner using 1/5 of the Complete Meal and 1/4 of the vegetables topped with 1/2 cup gravy.

### Betty Crocker Complete Meals: Herb Stuffing & Turkey Festive Dinner Style

| | |
|---|---|
| 1 package Betty Crocker Complete Meals Herb Stuffing and Turkey | 1/5 box serving 250 cal |
| 2 – 1 lb. bags frozen green beans | approx. 80 cal per 1/2 pound |
| 1 jar Heinz Fat Free Turkey Gravy | 20 cal per 1/4 cup |

Prepare turkey and stuffing meal according to directions. Steam vegetables in microwave. Assemble each 350 calorie dinner using 1/4 of the vegetables, 1/4 cup gravy and 1/5 of the turkey and stuffing meal.

### Betty Crocker Tuna Helper

| | |
|---|---|
| 1 package Betty Crocker Tuna Helper or Tuna Helper Creamy Parmesan | 160 cal per 1 cup serving |

2 bags frozen cut green beans or other vegetable of same calorie count
Kraft Fat Free grated Parmesan                    20 cal per serving

Prepare Tuna Helper according to directions. Microwave green beans and divide into 4 portions. Assemble each delicious 330 calorie dinner using one cup Helper and one portion of vegetables topped with one serving fat-free parmesan.

There is a plethora of Betty Crocker "Helper" meals, one better than the next which are naturals for your Festive dinner:

| | |
|---|---|
| Lasagna Bake | 270 cal for 1/5 box, prepared |
| Chicken and Potatoes Au Gratin | 270 cal for 1/5 box, prepared |
| Hamburger Helper Beef Pasta | 270 cal for 1 cup, prepared |
| Beef Stew | 260 cal for 1 cup, prepared |
| Beef Taco | 280 cal for 1 cup, prepared |
| Beef Teriyaki | 290 cal for 1 cup, prepared |
| Cheddar Melt | 310 cal for 1 cup, prepared |
| Chili Macaroni | 290 cal for 1 cup, prepared |
| Spaghetti | 280 cal for 1 cup, prepared |
| Fettuccini Alfredo | 300 cal for 1 cup, prepared |
| Creamy Parmesan | 300 cal for 1 cup, prepared |
| Lasagna | 270 cal for 1 cup, prepared |
| Pizza Pasta and Cheese Topping | 280 cal per 1 cup, prepared |
| Stroganoff | 290 cal for 1 cup, prepared |
| Ravioli with Cheese Topping | 310 cal for 1 cup, prepared |
| Rice Oriental | 280 cal for 1 cup, prepared |
| Salisbury | 280 cal for 1 cup, prepared |

Prepare Helper meal according to package directions. Choose a compatible vegetable with a calorie count of 80 calories per half pound, or less. You might choose mushrooms, zucchini, broccoli, cauliflower or green beans for example. The vegetables can be used as a bed for the Helper or they can be dressed with fat-free Promise margarine, Heinz fat-free gravy or Walden Farms calorie free salad dressing. Tasty and easy!

## Double Cheeseburger

| | |
|---|---|
| 1 1/2 light hamburger buns, toasted | 120 cal total |
| 2 Boca Burgers | 70 cal each |
| 1 slice Smart Beat fat free American cheese | 25 cal each |
| Walden Farms Fat-Free Thousand Island dressing | |
| 1/2 cup shredded Lettuce | |
| 2–3 slices of pickle | |
| 1 tsp. finely diced onion | |

Remove a thin slice of the top of the half hamburger bun. This will be the middle bun on your burger. Toast the half bun and the whole bun in the toaster until golden. Microwave the Boca Burgers according to package.

Assemble burger, from bottom in the following order: bottom bun, 1 tablespoon dressing, 1/2 teaspoon onion, 1/4 cup lettuce, 1 slice cheese, 1 burger, middle bun, more dressing, 1/2 teaspoon onion, 1/4 cup lettuce, pickles, second burger, top of bun. Reminiscent of a fast food favorite but only 315 calories, 340 if you'd like to add another slice of cheese. You can have a mini bag of Funyuns Onion Flavored rings (110 cal per 3/4 ounce bag) and a tall Diet Coke to complete your very American style meal for a total of 435 calories.

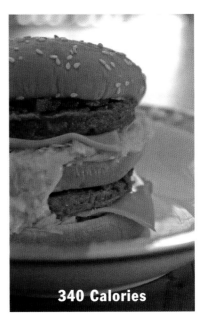

**340 Calories**

*Double Cheeseburger*

## Reuben Sandwich

| | |
|---|---|
| 2 slices Light Rye | 80 cal |
| 2 slices fat-free Swiss cheese | 60 cal |
| 3 oz. Budigg corned beef | 120 cal |
| Sauerkraut (14 oz. can) | |

The fattening Reuben sandwich is usually made with 2 slices of rye bread (160 calories), 2 slices of Swiss Cheese (160 calories) and 3 ounces of fatty corned beef (250 calories) and sauerkraut. That's over 600 calories! My Reuben, made with Light Rye (80 calories), 2 slices of fat-free Swiss cheese (60 calories) and 3 ounces of Budigg corned beef (120 calories) and sauerkraut comes to a delicious 260 calories.

## Chicken Cordon Bleu

| | |
|---|---|
| 1 1/4 pounds chicken breast cutlets | |
| 3 slices turkey ham, | 67 cal total |
| or 2 oz. any very thin sliced deli style ham | |
| 1 cup fat-free chicken broth | 10 cal |
| 3 oz. part skim mozzarella cheese | |
| 3 Tbs. grated Romano cheese | |

Divide chicken breasts, cheese and ham into six portions each. Flatten each chicken breast portion and top with one portion of ham and mozzarella cheese. Roll chicken breast and place seam side down in baking pan. Pour broth over chicken breasts and top with Romano cheese. Bake at 425 degrees for fifteen minutes. 233 calories for each of 6 chicken breasts.

## Vegetable Terrine

| | |
|---|---|
| 2 country refrigerator biscuits (to be used as bottom) | 100 cal |
| 1 jar junior baby food carrots | 60 cal |
| 1/2 of a 10 oz. package frozen spinach, thawed | 35 cal |
| 1 cup frozen mashed turnips | 50 cal |
| 1 cup mashed squash | 55 cal |
| 1 jar junior baby food sweet potato or peas | 120 cal |
| 1 package instant chicken broth | 5 cal |

Place biscuits in bottom of a loaf pan. Blend vegetables together and pour onto biscuits. Sprinkle with chicken broth and bake at 350 degrees for 20 minutes. 450 calories for entire recipe. Serves 4.

## Simple Lo Mein

|  |  |
|---|---|
| 2 packages (8 ounces each) Shirataki noodles (the kind made without tofu) | 50 cal per 8 oz. bag |
| 2 Tbs. House of Tsang Classic Stir Fry sauce | 25 cal per Tbs. |

Rinse noodles very thoroughly under cold water. Heat in boiling water or microwave, drain and pat dry with paper towel. Toss hot noodles in Stir fry sauce. 150 calories for a delicious lunch.


# SIDES & SAUCES

## Boo's Hollandaise

1 – 12 ounce container Light 'n Lively, fat-free cottage cheese
1 tsp. butter extract

Combine ingredients in a blender. Blend at low speed, stopping to scrape down sides until smooth. 215 calories for entire recipe.

## White Sauce (For Chipped Beef, creamed Chicken etc.)

1 Tbs. cake flour
2 tsp. cornstarch
4 Tbs. powdered skim milk
1 pack butter buds sprinkle
1 1/2 cups water
2 generous pinches salt
1 generous pinch pepper

Dissolve 2 teaspoons of cornstarch in 1/4 of the *cold* water. Put dissolved cornstarch, other 1 1/4 cups of water, powdered milk, pepper, and butter buds in pot. Cook on low, do not let simmer. Add flour a couple of pinches at a time stirring constantly. When all flour is incorporated and the mixture has been cooking 15 minutes turn the heat up to medium, add salt and let simmer. Keep stirring until the mixture starts to thicken. Note: it will continue to thicken as it cools. 145 calories total

## Spinach Souffle

| | |
|---|---|
| 2 – 10 oz. packages frozen chopped spinach, thawed | 140 cal total |
| 1 – 8 oz. carton Egg Beaters | 120 cal |
| 1/2 tsp. onion salt | |
| 1/4 tsp. grated nutmeg | |
| 1 cup evaporated skim milk | 90 cal |

Blend all ingredients in mixing bowl. Pour into a one quart baking dish and bake at 350 degrees for one hour. 350 calories for entire soufflé.

## Butter Buds Clam Sauce

| | |
|---|---|
| 1 – 4 oz. can minced clams | 50 cal |
| 1 Tbs. parsley | |
| 1 Tbs. garlic, minced | |
| 3 Tbs. plus 1 tsp. reconstituted Butter Buds | 40 cal |

Stir over low flame until hot. 90 calories for entire recipe. Create a Festive meal by boiling and draining one ounce pasta (210 cal), steaming 1/2 pound broccoli florets (80 cal), and tossing the sauce, broccoli and pasta together. 390 calories. Or use Shirataki noodles for lower calories.

## Broiled Tomato with Basil (side dish)

| | |
|---|---|
| 1 medium tomato, cut in half crosswise | 25 cal |
| Dried Basil | |

Sprinkle tomato with basil and broil until bubbly. 2 servings, 25 calories each.

# CHAPTER 13

# Since You've Got It, Flaunt It!

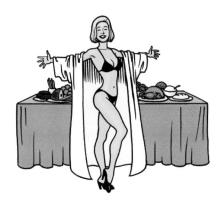

IF YOU FOLLOW MY GUIDANCE and serve the wonder new foods you'll know soon enough if your guests are impressed or are turned off by them. Benefit by my experience of the last decades. I told you the story of my first venture into the field. I hosted a benefit for autistic children. I announced to my guests that I was experimenting with these foods and felt them to be wonder foods. I was using the early Louis Rich creations of turkey-based ham, salami etc, as hors d'oeuvres. To my surprise, their response ranged from approving to enthusiastic. I then proceeded to have weekly tastings of low fat chili and Egg Foo Yung. People began to seek after invitations to my tastings. The positive comments outweighed the negative by a ratio of at least 5 to 1. This ratio would be good if I served ChateauBriand and Baked Alaska. The first time you serve your guests the miracle foods from your pantry you may well be nervous. Take the plunge and **tell them what you are serving them**. Assert that some of the cold cuts are varied forms of turkey, and that the cream cheese, sour cream, mayonnaise, and salad dressing are fat-free. You may well be delighted by their reactions.

The most flagrant fat eater is conscious of the need for lean foods for the sake of his heart and weight and general health. He may not yet be strong enough to serve these wonder foods in his own home. He may not be able to choose them if they are offered at restaurants. He will, however, be grateful to you for forcing him to do what every sane person wants to do. He will be grateful to you for forcing him to eat these low calorie wonder new foods.

Extend this sanity into the area of soft drinks. The most overt insanity of our nutritional world is the use of high fructose sweetened soda. Advertising is effective. Pretty girls have been drinking "Classic Coke" on TV for years. The only really difficult times I've had in serving my foods have been in the area of carbonated drinks. I've had guests who would not drink "that horrible no cal stuff." In spite of the fact that, in one taste test after another, the subject could not tell the "artificial" sweetener from the natural, and often they prefer the "artificial," they are conditioned to know that "natural" sugar is good and "artificial sweetener" is bad. I have tried to point out that some of the new artificial sweeteners are simply intensified forms of natural sugar. "My mind is made up. Don't confuse me with the facts!" Those imprinted with the sexiness of Classic Coke are lost causes. I've stopped arguing with them. I now provide these special guests with a bottle containing seventeen teaspoons of sugar per serving. I have learned when I can fight and when fighting is hopeless. Let them eat sugar.

# CHAPTER 14

# "I Can't Believe I Ate the Whole Thing"

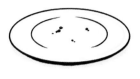

THE SAD HISTORY OF DIETING is that all previous diets were hunger diets. Dieting was associated with cottage cheese, an eighth of a melon and some Jell-O. The dieters lost some weight when they began the regimen but gained it back with additional pounds for good measure. There were warning voices along the way. Many medical authorities have emphasized the importance of the insulin cycle. The dieter ate a piece of fruit and eight ounces of skim milk. His insulin cycle spiked from the nourishment. Because the nourishment was so sparse and so infrequent the insulin level plummeted and, sooner or later, the dieter had to binge in the classic pig-out.

I have based my program on the converse of this premise.
By now the major medical authorities agree that:

## HUNGER LEADS TO WEIGHT GAIN.

Since hunger leads to weight gain, the converse is evident:

## FULLNESS LEADS TO WEIGHT LOSS.

The nutrition cycle of the bear is but one of the many, many examples in nature that buttress this principle. Our object then is to reverse the old association of hunger leading to weight loss, and to follow the truth that we now know, fullness leads to weight loss. My whole program is directed to this end.

I have already discussed long range food shopping. Fill your freezer, pantry and refrigerator with tasty low calorie filling foods. Now I want to devote some thought to the act of fullness nourishing. Reverse the old eighth of a melon and six ounces of skim milk feeling with the Festive program of 5 1/2 cups of Pop Secret butter flavored popcorn. EAT THE WHOLE BAG. In place of half cup of regular Jell-O eat the whole package of Festive sugar free Jell-O. Again, I repeat, EAT THE WHOLE THING.

Good begets good. Focusing on volume eating leads to loss of weight and also to robust health. Fats and proteins are calorie rich. It is the vegetables and greens that are low in calories and lead to the desired fullness. The Asian body has long been considered the ideal of slenderness. Before our Western influence took effect a fat Asian was an anomaly. The Asian lived on vegetables with rice and fish. He knew little of the cholesterol and heart disease that plague our society. His diet is the one we seek at the Chinese restaurant where vegetables are made to feel fatty and delicious soaked in cornstarch. The Asian made his bulk diet tastier than our high calorie diets.

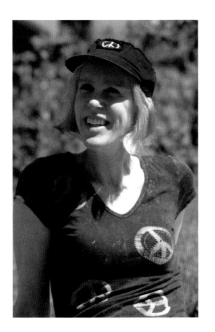

*My 55th Birthday*

I have developed many delicious, low calorie, filling vegetable and greens dishes over the years. For lunch on this wintry day I had a brick of cauliflower, which I boiled in four cups of chicken broth made with Herb-Ox bullion. I garnished it with slices of a fat-free hot dog. This monster stew with steaming broth, vegetable and meat filled me physically and emotionally. I have made many variations of this Festive stew with various vegetables such as a frozen brick of broccoli, green beans or spinach. My favorite soups for these Festive meals are Campbell's Chicken Noodle O's, Manhattan clam chowder, and the many Progresso and Healthy Choice soups with pasta, all of which are less than two hundred calories for the entire can. In warmer weather I concentrate on a monster chef's salad made with cucumber, tomato and other greens garnished with the thin sliced Hillshire farm meats, bacon bits, fat-free cheese and, of course tons of our calorie free dressings. Try some of my Festive dinners made of a Lean Cuisine frozen entrée and an entire brick of vegetables topped with one of the low or no calorie dressings or sauces and you may find that you have to work to finish the 400 calorie feast.

In a similar vein I find soups to be a most desirable food. Along with my Irish and English ancestry I must have some Slavic background. Soups were peasant foods. Throw whatever you have from the garden or leftover from previous meals into some water and you have the soup of the country in which you live. Bouillabaisse was the Marseille garbage repository of leftover shellfish, vegetables and potatoes. Russian serfs were literally slaves of their lords. They lived on borscht and black bread. Part of the beet harvest was fed as slop for the pigs. The peasants boiled the other part of the beet harvest into borscht. In New York the Russian Tea Room charged five dollars for a cup of the same borscht.

I loathe beggardom. I revel in plenty. Soup is a prime answer to my need. Instead of diets offering half a cup of string beans, I've urged you to "eat the whole thing." In the wintertime boil the block of broccoli or cauliflower in a broth made with chicken or beef or vegetable bullion. In the summer time chill the soup and add fat-free sour cream. The peasant in you will triumph and you will become slim, trim and Slavic.

You must create your own dishes featuring substantial quantities of food that are delicious and low calorie. Use the wonder foods that I emphasize. 99% fat-free bologna and hot dogs and bacon bits are basic garnishes. Eat the whole bag of "buttered popcorn." Eat the whole box of sugar free pudding made with water instead of milk, (the taste is identical). Eat the whole box of sugar free Jell-O topped with whipped cream. Be lavish and generous to your taste buds and to your digestive system and to your psyche. Enjoy my fullness program and the slenderness it will bring.

# CHAPTER 15

# Use Your Noodle

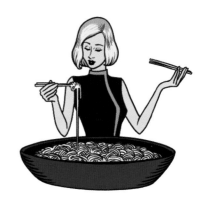

FESTIVE EATING is based on arithmetic. The trick is to prepare the most lavish meal with the lowest calories. It is a fact of my program that you can gorge shamefully on rich food that makes your body actually slim down.

The light breads are revolutionary. They are half the calories of standard bread and are actually richer in fiber. Imagine eating two full slices which equal the calories of one of the old fashioned slices. The bread equation, however, is eclipsed by the Shirataki equation. Pasta is as much a staple of diet as bread or rice. All these staples have been high in calories. The half calorie bread was the first breakthrough. The new pasta is not a breakthrough, it is a supernova. The mathematical ratio of old fashioned pasta to the new Shirataki noodles is an awesome 210 to 40 — less than a fifth of the calories. For bread to be that impressive the new slices would have to be only 13 calories instead of the present 80. Even more unbelievable is the simple Shirataki noodle made without tofu. This awesome product weighs in at less than half the calories of the tofu version. It approaches the negative caloric value of celery. The energy required to eat a stalk of celery burns more calories than the celery contributes to the body. You lose weight as you eat. This yam noodle approaches this ideal.

With this arithmetic on our side the wise thing is to make the Shirataki noodle as important a part of this diet as your imagination will allow. Whole books have been written on pasta recipes since Marco Polo brought pasta from China to Italy. I have a good number of pasta recipes in my collection. I haven't experimented fully with the Shirataki noodle because it is so new an addition to the American market. This incredible product is made up of tofu and yam flour. Glucommanan, the fat fighter, is a derivative of yam flour. I haven't yet mastered the details of how they take these two healthful ingredients and produce so rich a noodle that has so few calories. But don't look a gift horse in the mouth. Run, do not walk, to a grocer who carries Shirataki noodles. Before I found grocers who carried it I ordered it from Amazon.com. Start your personal experimentation with this marvelous product that is delicious, filling and UNBELIEVABLY LOW IN CALORIES.

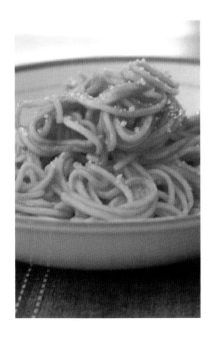

*Shirataki Noodles*

It took me a few trials to get the hang of preparing the noodles. They have to be rinsed, drained and heated. They should be eaten al dente — slightly firm. The angel hair pasta form of the noodle is my favorite. The slight firmness also makes the digestive process a longer one and keeps the feeling of fullness longer.

There is no end to the creative dishes with Shirataki noodles as their base. So far one of my favorites is macaroni and cheese and I make a cheese sauce for it based on corn starch and cheese flavored No More Naked Popcorn (the No More Naked Popcorn company has a great recipe for this in their brochure. I personally prefer the yellow cheddar over the white). I use the noodles as a base for Egg Foo Yung. The noodles cut the calories so sharply that I've opted to use whole eggs rather than Egg Beaters and still remained within the dinner calories.

As far as standard spaghetti and noodle dishes the ones I've enjoyed so far are: with spaghetti sauce and sausage, stroganoff, with white clam sauce, in tuna casserole, alfredo (Walden Farms no calorie), with Walden Farms scampi sauce, with our butter and parsley, and sprinkled with No More Naked Popcorn Parmesan & Garlic sprinkle. Use your own noodle to create your personal recipes.

I am sure that nuclear energy and space travel are wonderful creations of science. They pale however, when compared with this ultimate product of our scientific era — the Shirataki noodle.

# CHAPTER 16

# The Panacea — No-Calorie Salad Dressing

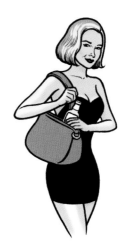

NO SELF-RESPECTING MAN, youngster or even woman will admit to a desire for lettuce, carrots and celery. We know the basic food groups of our society — hamburgers, hot dogs and pizza. The standard sit-com shows the mother trying to bribe the child to eat her vegetables at dinnertime. An acquaintance of mine told me that she sneaked a stalk of celery into the meatloaf so that the family would have a vegetable course.

Medical authorities hammer their refrain. Eat more basic fibrous food. The bran of whole wheat and brown rice is necessary for a myriad of reasons. The response of our fast food society is to consider catsup a vegetable because it has a tomato base (though it is mostly sugar).

This, then, is the challenge. I am not going to change the bad eating habits overnight. The addiction to fat is just that, an addiction. It has been demonstrated in laboratory tests that rats offered fat will eat more and more fat to the exclusion of normal food. The result on their health and weight is disastrous. Fat is an addiction and addictions are stronger than the natural desire for health.

This is the dilemma we face. We have trained ourselves to eat fat to a point where we've forgotten that the basic human diet has been cereal and greens. The obsession with fat has overcome our intelligence. We know it is bad for us but we are ever more addicted to our basic food groups, fatty pizza, hamburgers and hot dogs. This pernicious trend was given quasi-medical support by the teachings of the once famous Dr. Atkins.

I could think of no way of solving this problem were it not for the miracle new foods which most good homemakers overlook. I know of no woman in my circle of friends who has a bottle of no calorie salad dressing in her pantry. This is the irony of our society.

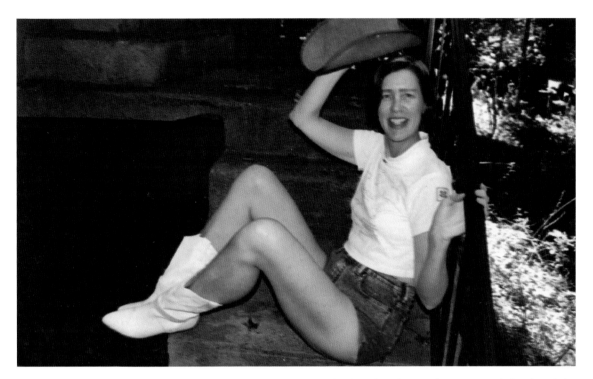

We have the answer to our dilemma — the desire for fat and our need for health. The new salad dressings are based on cornstarch and gums and other fibers. They give us the texture of fat and the taste of fat with little or no fat in them. The balkiest football husband or crankiest child will relish vegetables and salad soaked in tasty, creamy dressing. By pulling the blinders from her eyes, the conscientious mother could now serve her family the foods that she knows they should have with dressings that are low or 0 in calories. Her dilemma would be gone. She now has a nifty solution to her problem, which her family will love. Until now she knew that she could have her family eat the salads and vegetables they need if she soaked them in regular salad dressing or butter. She couldn't think the thought because it would be self-defeating. The salad dressings she knew were 70 to 120 calories for the minimal 2 tablespoon serving. They might as well be eating fatty hamburgers. Until now there seemed to her to be no way out of the dilemma.

The last two decades have seen the development of a whole array of new salad dressings. The mother can choose from 0 calorie to 5 to 25 to 40 calories for the two tablespoon serving. This is in contrast to the standard 70 to 120 for a serving of the standard salad dressing. The possibilities are staggering. I recommend the creamy 0 calorie Walden Farms line among others. These are also available in packets which can be carried along when you go out to eat. I eat my salads and vegetables dripping with creamy dressings. The calories are minimal and the taste is better than the fatty taste of the standard products.

I hope this book jolts the American woman out of her rut. I love my grandmother very much but I don't use the corset or the bustle. I also rarely use the oven; most of my food is prepared in the microwave. Why I should use her crummy, fatty salad dressings is beyond me. Her terms of "chemical" and "unnatural" are terms based on ignorance. All foods are chemicals; everything that exists in nature is natural. I have told you repeatedly that fat substitutes like modified food starch, xanthan gum and cellulose gel are either perfectly harmless or actually nutritious. If you have any of the old fashioned prejudices that stop you from using gifts of science like low calorie corn-starch instead of fat, snap out of it. Alexander cut the Gordian knot by slashing it in two with his sword. Bob Newhart portrayed a shrink who solved all his clients' problems with two words. When they described their destructive habits he responded, "So, don't." You know, vaguely, that you are avoiding the new salad dressings for antiquated reasons. You are acting ignorantly by blindly following the prejudices of your grandmother. "So, don't."

There is in addition another whole world of uses for these new salad dressings. I can't keep up with the statistics about eating out. Just a few years ago the American family ate a third of its meals outside the home. That percentage keeps climbing. I suspect it will soon be more than half the meals that are eaten outside the home. You the diner are trapped. Good restaurants serve the standard fatty dressings and garnishes. The salads you eat in the restaurant give you the fiber you need but they also stuff you with destructive calories. The new dressings offer the dream solution to the problem. They give you the salad dressing taste and the fiber with zero calories.

It is unthinkable to bring food into a restaurant. If you brought an entrée or side dish to eat into a restaurant you would be using the restaurant's facilities while eating your own food. The restaurant would go broke. There are two exceptions to this rule. One exception is the custom of bringing your own wine into the restaurant. If there is a special wine you like you hand the bottle to the sommelier. He serves it and charges you a corkage fee. You get the wine you like and the restaurant makes out well. The other exception to the general rule is salad dressing. Even the fussiest restaurateur knows that he has clients who for health or other reasons need a certain salad dressing — which the restaurant may not offer. The client who brings his own salad dressing still pays for the salad. The salad dressing is not part of the cost of the meal. One can openly bring his bottle of salad dressing and place it on the table for all to see. This, then, opens the door to whole new possibilities of having the best of both worlds.

The dressings I love are perfect for salad, but they are also great for vegetables and even for entrées. Suddenly the option is not whether to have your vegetable order either steamed and tasteless or covered in fatty butter. That same bottle of salad dressing standing in the middle of the table can be poured onto your vegetables or fish or other entrée so that you have the delicious fatty taste with few or no calories. No longer are you stuck behind the false dilemma of either eating blah greens or blah vegetables or broiled, dry, sauce-less entrees or making them fattening by covering them with fat and calories. You can now eat in the restaurant of your choice and delight in dishes that now will be both delicious, low calorie and free of fat. Enjoy!

# CHAPTER 17

# All the Rest is Gravy

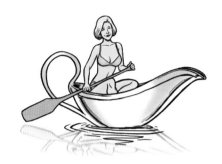

MEAT IS THE LUXURY FOOD of the wealthy. Oliver Twist asked for more gruel. Later the beadle found that the orphanage had fed him scraps of meat that the dog wouldn't eat. Even so, it was meat and the honorable beadle was horrified that an orphan should get any kind of meat. When the lower classes did get meat, it was often in the form of humble pie. The term "eating humble pie" connotes to us apologetic kissing of your adversary's toe. There was however a food called humble pie. When the deer was cut up after the hunt the gentry ate the loin and the other good cuts of meat. The entrails and the other inedible parts were wrapped with dough and fed to the humble folk. This was humble pie.

The consumption of meat was the mark of wealth but it had its price. Royal portraits show Henry VIII eating his chunk of fatty meat while suffering gout, obesity and the other plagues of the wealthy. Eating "the fat of the land" had its price. To this day the value of beef depends on the marbling. Prime rib is the fattiest and the costliest. The more fat, the higher the grade of beef. Kobe beef comes from steers fed on beer. Personal attendants massage the animal till the fat enters every part of the meat. It, too, is very costly.

This tradition of meat as being a luxury and penalized by fat and cholesterol is our heritage to this day. An important dinner features Prime Rib, the beef with the most fat. Intelligent people and the best chefs still use only gravy made out of drippings. "Drippings" is a polite word for liquid fat. We are still faced with the choice of being healthy or of eating a piece of prime rib with globs of chunk fat.

I can think of no greater gift to prepare a young bride for her future as the family chef than a jar or can of fat-free gravy. This gravy has been on the grocery shelves for at least a decade. One would imagine this is the only gravy an intelligent person would use. Its taste is exactly the same as the fatty gravy but it is based on cornstarch instead of drippings. Why there are still holdouts who insist on the fatty gravy I don't know. With obesity indicators rising sharply it's hard to imagine why the various brands of fat-free gravy are still shunned by many intelligent people.

I have wracked my brain over this anomaly. How can perfectly lovely, bright young mothers whose children have weight problems continue to feed them gravy made of fat and flour when there is Heinz and other low- or no-cal gravies on hand. The only answers I could come up with was that good food was always elaborate to prepare and had to be fatty. From the beginning of our culture upper classes ate "high on the hog."

Confusing good cuisine with elaborate preparation of fatty meats goes back to the origin of our culture. William conquered England in 1066 and for centuries the court spoke only French. The peasant Saxons spoke a Germanic language. We therefore have two words for each subject. The poor "hause" is German, a palatial home is a French "maison", or mansion. The poor farmer dealt with the schwein, (swine), the wealthy noble ate the (French) bacon. The farmer dealt with the German "kuh"(cow), the noble ate the French boeuf (beef).

This is the tradition we inherit. A fine, noble meal must be elaborately prepared by staffs of chiefs (chefs) and based on complex, fatty recipes. Anything simple is peasant fare and is unworthy. My analysis also accounted for the recipe books we all have on our shelves. One of the new recipe books that I bought has 600 recipes. Each recipe has between eight and twenty ingredients. They all require "2 tablespoons of fresh chopped chives, 2 ounces of tarragon vinegar, etc." My colleagues and I tried to follow one of the recipes. It involved marinating four ounces of fillet of sole in a marinade made up of five ingredients. The ingredients cost us $38 and the meal took three hours to assemble. The only way we could account for this penchant for complexity is that we still suffer from the heritage that equates good food with complexity and expense. These foods take six times as long to prepare as to eat.

I want all of you to raise your hands and become brand new brides. Go home tonight and feed your family as a modern young princess with no memory of old prejudices. Fat-free gravy fits all my criteria. It is delicious, filling, readily available and very low-calorie. The only reason not to use it is that you are stuck in outdated tradition, or that you don't like health for yourself and your family members. There is simply no down-side to the use of fat-free gravies. The multitude of their uses is self-evident. Enjoy.

# CHAPTER 18

# *Hidden Hungers*

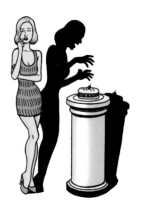

HIDDEN HUNGER IS OFTEN A FACTOR in causing obesity. Dogs eat mud because they need some mineral found in the mud. Our bodily needs drive us to eat many bananas if we need potassium, no matter how much they add to our weight. We may have no idea why we are eating the bananas. We may not even like bananas, but we have to eat them because of what nutritionists label "hidden hunger."

Hidden hungers are inexorable forces. Fighting them simply doesn't work. We have to recognize them and fulfill them. The job involves you. You have to be aware of personal cravings. You must spot them and try to fulfill them. The range is so wide that no nutritionist can specify what particular need or needs your metabolism requires. Nutritionists can help, but you are an essential part of spotting these hidden hungers.

We have dealt with the prime overt hunger, which is the need for sweetness. This need was a disastrous cause of obesity. There simply were no sweeteners that did not cause obesity. I've told you how my own experience in seeking a non-caloric sweetener was such an uphill challenge. Saccharine was out, cyclamates were banned, the first non-fattening soft drink, Tab, was hardly drinkable. Now we have the blessing of multiple no-cal sweeteners to fulfill this primary hunger for sweetness.

Another overt hunger is the desire for salt. The desire for salt is an artificial one and it is pernicious. You could live a healthy life if you never lifted a salt shaker. The salt found naturally in ordinary food is more than ample for your physical needs. It is the addition of salt to prepared food that habituates us to the use of additional salt. Potato chips, canned soups and restaurant food are made more enticing by pouring on the salt. The habit of pouring salt is an acquired one. People with heart conditions soon learn that other taste enhancers can do the job beautifully with no danger to their physical well-being. Horseradish and peppers are common taste enhancers that can cut down the use of salt. Nu-Salt and Salt-Sense are among the many new products that cut down your use of this pernicious, high blood pressure inducing condiment. In short order you will think of these substitutes as "salt" and you will be healthier for the replacement.

Another common hidden hunger is the need for the mouth-feel of crunchiness. A woman I know went on a bland liquid diet. She cried to me,"I'd give anything for a crunchy candy bar but that would be breaking my diet." There is a low calorie classic food that fills this need to a "T." It is that ancient staple of the Indians, popcorn. Corn was cultivated in Mexico seven thousand years ago and ears of popping corn were found in a bat cave in New Mexico and are thought to be over five thousand years old. When Columbus arrived in the West Indies the natives sold popcorn to his crew. When the Pilgrims landed at Plymouth Rock, they were greeted by Native Americans wearing popcorn necklaces. Popcorn was the adornment on Grandfather's Christmas tree before our era of tinsel and lights. We Americans already eat more popcorn than anyone else in the world — about 70 quarts a year, but we still don't think of it as a basic food.

It is high time that we took this marvelous food out of its category of optional snack food for movie-goers or television snackers. The small bag of Pop Secret Light yields almost six cups and totals only 100 calories. It fits beautifully in my criteria of foods that are tasty, low calorie and filling. Now, add to these benefits the unique crunchy mouth feel. No dieter has to go astray eating caloric chips and candy bars in his hidden hunger for the crunch mouth feel.

Popcorn is an example of how the new foods supplement each other. In olden days popcorn was heavily caloric. Air popped corn tasted like chopped cardboard. The theater owner poured tons of butter onto it to make it palatable. 100 calorie a tablespoon butter made the snack caloric. It also made it soggy and impaired its crunch mouth feel. With the advent of artificial butter flavor, Molly McButter (in cheese and butter flavor), Butter Buds in the shaker and other low calorie, rich buttery-tasting additives we can now have our popcorn and eat it too. The latest of the new toppings are the No More Naked Popcorn shakers providing eleven new flavors for popcorn. Excellent!  My epicure friends have sweetened the popcorn with Equal or Splenda and cinnamon. Extremists eat it spicy with chili seasoning, curry powder or paprika. My own favorite is Molly McButter cheese sprinkle. All these additions give us our crunchy, low calorie product with no down side. Take this delicacy out of the category of movie and TV snack fare and make it a staple of your family diet as I have. Its crunchiness is a basic weapon in the battle against the pig out.

Another hidden hunger that leads to pig-outs is the desire for the fatty mouth feel. This common hidden hunger can be satisfied with healthful foods that are low calorie. The one that I find most satisfying and with the widest range of uses is the much neglected cornstarch. You all know about its properties because you have eaten in Chinese restaurants. Chinese food is rated by most nutritionists as the most healthful of cuisines. The secret of Chinese cuisine is cornstarch. Chinese vegetables give you the fatty mouth feel with no fat in them thanks to their sauce based on cornstarch. One popular soup at a Chinese restaurant is egg drop soup. It is a low calorie dish made of chicken broth, shreds of egg and of course the ever-present cornstarch.

Cornstarch makes even the most threatening of desserts accessible calorically. The caloric demon of desserts is pie. Piecrust is full of butter. A small slice of pie is around three hundred calories. In my Festive desserts I offer you sinfully rich phyllo tarts stuffed with fruit filling made according to the description below. This Festive dessert miracle is achieved through the use of our sweeteners, readily available 18 calorie Athens brand frozen mini pastry shells, and of course, our trusty old cornstarch. One of my favorite creations is a "Napoleon" made with sugar-free cheesecake mousse. My guests are blown away when I tell them that this super-rich dessert is just 35 calories. An additional plus to this taste sensation is that it is easy to make. Blend the mousse with cold water and pour it into the puff pastry shells. The shells can also be filled with sugar free chocolate, pumpkin, vanilla and strawberry mousse made the same way.

Another gourmet treasure is pie filled with apple or cherry filling sweetened with Splenda and, of course, enriched with cornstarch. Lucky Leaf is one of my favorites. Comstock has always had sliced apples in water but required the addition of cornstarch and some of our sweetener. Just follow the directions for dissolving the cornstarch in water, mix with the apples in a pan and cook until thickened, then add sweetener to taste. This recipe can also be used with bags of frozen peaches, strawberries and blueberries. Comstock's new product is ready made apple pie filling, ready to use with only 245 calories for the entire 20 oz. can. Comstock also has a cherry pie filling sweetened with Splenda, 245 calories for the can. **You can have your pie and be slender too!**

Cornstarch is an ideal thickener. It is more effective calorie-wise than flour for gravies etc. It is better and more healthful than butter or other fats. This old-fashioned product should be a staple in your pantry. If you are adventuresome, read the simple directions on the use of Xanthan gum for similar purposes. Xanthan gum is available in health food stores.

In this category of varied mouth-feels we must feature the magic mushroom. We will now give you a list of all the foods in which mushrooms are not a valuable addition. These foods are coffee, chocolate syrup and ice cream. I am exaggerating, of course, but mushrooms have almost unlimited use. Whole cookbooks have been written on recipes based on mushrooms. They take on the taste of whatever food they garnish. They are perfect for meats, fish, eggs (quiche), as a meat substitute, in salad, etc. etc. In kosher restaurants that serve only dairy food they also serve "meat" dishes. Since the dietary law forbids them from using real meat the lamb chops and veal and other "meat' dishes are made of mushrooms. I have eaten these dishes and they are surprisingly good. You remember the old adage, "If it sounds too good to be true, it probably is." An exception to this rule is the versatile, delicious mushroom. Fresh mushrooms are only seven calories an ounce. Their cost is in line with other food costs. By making a habit of adding mushrooms to your food you will make your foods epicurean delights. Mushrooms give your food a fatty mouth- feel and add to the flavor of whatever dish they are in. An additional bonus is that they make you full with very low calories. They are one of my prized examples of low calorie filling food. Simply by adding mushrooms to your food you will lose calories and pounds. Make mushrooms a staple food in your diet.

There is nothing new under the sun. None of the ingredients or processes that I use is original to me: they have all been used before. The unique thing about my Fullness Program is my approach.

# CHAPTER 19

# The Medical Priority, "Get The Weight Off"

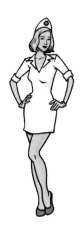

MANY OF US HAVE MULTIPLE HEALTH PROBLEMS. The fight against obesity should take priority over almost all other problems. A friend of mine is obese and at the same time he is a heavy smoker. His doctor wants him to stop smoking. The doctor told my friend, however, to keep smoking if that helped him get rid of his weight. Getting rid of that dangerous load of fat was more important than anything else, even if it meant continuing the curse of smoking.

You have to be dedicated to getting rid of your weight. You must not only follow my program but you must also give it priority. My Fullness Program is based on nature's getting rid of your fat for you once you truly feel full. You must analyze yourself. You know your own patterns of pigging out. Perhaps for you it was your need for the mouth-feel of crunchiness that made you eat that nut bar. Perhaps you needed a taste of fat which made you gulp that hot dog at the mall. Analyze the pitfalls and deal with them. Keeping full on minimal calories is the name of the game. Avoid the traps of pigging out on high calorie food. I have tried to provide for the various tastes and mouth feels in my menus. Nobody knows you like you know yourself. I write for a general audience. You must look out for number one, yourself.

As you understand my program of being full on low calorie food you become my partner and friend in following the program. Analyze yourself and be creative and original. Certainly it is good to get the benefit of fibers and vegetables etc, but THE IMPORTANT THING IS TO GET THE FAT OFF. You might find that you are hankering after sweets. Do as I did. There were times that I used up all my calories on sugar-free chocolate pudding and my Festive brownie. I remember making whole meals out of popcorn alone. There were times that I consciously went over my calories a little bit so as not to have a set-back with a major pig-out.

You must be passionate about getting the fat off. To that end you must understand the principals of my Fullness Program. Surely I'd like you to have the balanced diet in the menus I've outlined. Remember, though, that you are taking a multivitamin pill every day. Nothing dangerous will happen if you avoid pig-outs by meals of sweet or crunchiness. The pig-out perpetuates the fat, and it is the pig-out which must be avoided at all costs.

You will probably succeed in losing your weight by blindly following my Fullness Program. I would be happier and your weight loss will be even more certain if you follow my program with understanding as my partner and friend. Help me do it by analyzing yourself. Think through the temptations which might lead you to the destructive pig-out. Fashion your menu with the lowest calorie answers to the pig-out. Let us help each other to get that weight off BY ALMOST ANY MEANS. Everything in my program is subject to the overall command, "Plan your program to avoid the pig- out at any cost. Get the fat off."

## Despising Food or Worshipping Food

FOOD IS SO FUNDAMENTAL a fact of human life that it brings out the most extreme reactions. At one extreme there are those who belittle the role of dining and of food in our lives. Our Puritan ancestors taught that the enjoyment of food was sinful. This teaching still affects us. One of the French gourmet magazines featured a full page cartoon of an American Thanksgiving dinner. It showed the table spread with the most luxurious food. The diners were shoveling the food as they smoked, drank cocktails, and watched the football game on television. They focused on everything but the delicious food spread before them. This shameful disregard of the beauty of dining is one of the less attractive traits of many Americans. It is evident at feast times but also at the fast food outlets which make up a huge part of our nutritional lives. I have been vocal in my feelings about those who abuse fast foods. It takes twenty minutes for the digestive process to register on the brain. Finishing the Whopper in seven minutes invites obesity. The diner has finished the food long before his mind registers that he has even eaten. He is a prime candidate for the pig-out.

At the other extreme are the dilettante gourmets. In my years in the food business I have come across many of these worshippers who make food and wine their gods. I would not resent them if they kept to themselves. With many of them however, their biggest kick is to put down those who are not of their religion. "You know, my dear, she actually served store bought bread at her dinner party." "Can you imagine, she served white wine unchilled?" I find these self-styled authorities to be the clowns in the field of nutrition. This "in group" equates culinary success with following their particular superstitions and with the amount of work they have expended and the amount of money they have spent.

There is a story of the man who asked his baker to prepare a cake in the shape of the letter E. You can make the story as long and as detailed as you like. When the customer came to pick up the cake he had to correct the order. The baker had made the cake as an italic E instead of a gothic E. When the customer came back for the corrected cake it turned out that it was Belgian chocolate instead of Swiss chocolate. You can go on and on about the decorations and the fillings etc. Finally, after a dozen tries the customer found the cake to be absolutely right. The baker asked, "Where shall I deliver it sir?" The customer answered, "No thanks, I'll just eat it here."

This artificiality about complexity for its own sake has filtered down to recipes for daily cooking. Slim·Fast was aimed to the mass market. A brochure was included with their products. One suggested recipe demanded six ounces of fish marinated in various oils and herbs. This recipe called for hours of shopping and work, dozens of dirty dishes and a large sum of money to make a meal. Can you imagine a normal housewife taking care of her kids or coming from work and going through this ordeal of shopping and elaborate food preparation? I couldn't help thinking of the fellow with the cake in the shape of an E. Unfortunately, this is not a humorous subject to the dieter. She feels that she has to go through all these convolutions to prepare a proper meal. One of my hopes is to counter these dilettantes and to offer valid recipes that are rich in their simplicity.

I have nothing but good to say about people who take an interest in herbs. Certainly they are entitled to their hobby. Our country is full of subcultures. There are magazines coming out monthly devoted to snowboarding and Volkswagens and spices. It's fine to have a hobby. It is pretentious to claim that this hobby makes one superior. A couple I know suffered a very difficult divorce. One of the causes of anguish was the division of the herbs that they'd gathered over the years. I would bet my bottom dollar that these creatures couldn't tell canned pepper from fresh ground pepper on their salads if they were blindfolded. This myth that hard work and expense create good food is just that — a myth.

An extreme of this pretentious artiness is the wine culture. Wine dates back to the earliest civilizations. When Noah landed after the flood the first thing that he did was to plant a vineyard. Since human waste was used for fertilizing crops water was a dangerous drink. We still know about the danger of drinking water in Mexico which can cause diarrhea — Montezuma's Revenge.

French and Italian children drink wine from infancy. It is a wonderful drink. Aficionados have every right to study the brands and to choose their favorites. The shame is that there are people who take these self styled authorities seriously. Fish calls for white wine? This is as stupid as saying that hamburger calls for Pepsi Cola and pizza calls for Coca Cola. The wine you like is the right wine. Anyone who tells you different is a joker.

I know one of these preachers who had the saving grace to laugh at his own social circle. They would faint with shock at the thought of serving champagne in other than the proper champagne flute etc. This fellow had a cabinet lined with black velvet. He bought various glasses at garage sales and put them in the cabinet. His friends would "ting" these dime store glasses and comment on them. He would respond with a straight face, "You are right that it is leaded glass but I'm not sure if it's Tuscany or Florence." Yes, he could laugh at these poseurs with their pretenses about wine goblets but he was religious in his devotion to the fact that only this wine must be drunk with this food etc. etc.

I had an experience along these lines. After college I lived in a high-rise apartment for a year. I often came home at the same time as a neighboring tenant and we sometimes found ourselves sharing the same elevator. He always carried 2 bottles of champagne for himself and guests. He confided in me that the cost was ruinous to him. I suggested that he buy a decent sauterne and pour it into one of the carbon dioxide siphons which is used to make soda water. I told him to fill the goblets in the kitchen and no one would ever tell the difference. He would have champagne at a fraction of the cost. Our little plot succeeded and he saved a ton of money. Incidentally, champagne is not the name of a drink, it is the name of a place. Sparkling wine made in the French province of Champagne is the only sparkling wine that has the right to be called Champagne. Sparkling wine made from grapes grown immediately outside the province can't be called Champagne. It is identical to Champagne, without the Champagne name and sells for a fraction of the price.

I don't enjoy lambasting these food and wine lovers. I do so only to stress the point that work and money are not necessary to superb dining. My friends and I have turned out marvelous meals with little effort and little cost. The prejudice that these creatures have established is hurting the nutrition of our country. The average woman simply can't "marinate six ounces of fish with chopped chives etc, etc." She then feels that she has to give up and serve her family second rate, fattening meals. This is simply not the truth. One part of my job is to discredit those who claim that leisure and wealth are needed for fine cooking. The other part of my job is to offer delicious, inexpensive menus that offer meals far better than the pretentious ones.

## Less Sleep = More Weight

I'VE QUOTED our government's pronouncement that obesity is a greater threat to us than heart disease and the other major illnesses combined. Now various branches of medicine are contributing insights to the causes of the plague. A recent study featured in national publications was the correlation of sleep patterns with obesity. The study showed correlation between the amount or lack of sleep and hunger patterns. They showed an example of one young man who was deprived of sleep over a matter of days. His rate of weight gain correlated exactly with the amount of his sleep deprivation. The doctor's explanation was that lack of sleep inhibits leptin, which makes the body experience fullness. At the same time this sleep deprivation intensifies secretion of gherlin, which makes the body crave food. Thus the person who is not getting enough sleep has an accelerator on his hunger pangs and the brakes are on his feelings of fullness. Americans have been sleeping less in the same period that obesity has burgeoned. As part of your program of fullness make normal sleep patterns a routine part of your activity.

# CHAPTER 20

# The Roadblocks We Overcame

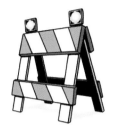

NOW THAT MY FULLNESS PROGRAM IS LAUNCHED I would like to share with you some of the whim whams I experienced during the development process. A major one was the feeling of "otherness" from the mainstream of nutritional thinking. There have been diets since olden times. These diets run the gamut of approaches to weight loss but there is one thing they all teach: LIMIT THE AMOUNTS OR KINDS OF FOOD YOU EAT AND YOU WILL LOSE WEIGHT. In other words, be hungry and you might become slender. I felt completely out of step with the mainstream of nutritional and dietary authorities. I felt out of step, so I felt that I might be wrong.

It was my feeling that the hunger approach is fruitless, but it is hard to buck the unanimous outlook of so many diets over so long a period of history. There is a story of a soldier's mother watching a parade of returning troops. She said proudly, "There were thousands of soldiers in the parade, but everyone was out of step except my Johnny." I felt that I was Johnny. How can I be right and everyone else wrong? But perhaps Johnny *was* right and it was the thousands of other soldiers who were out of step. Since the hundreds of diets based on hunger haven't worked, might it not be time to think of an opposite approach to nutrition that might work?

How can we be the first to create a fullness program for weight control? Our program is simple. All the authorities agree that hunger makes you hang on to weight. You discipline yourself to be on this diet or that one and you hold on as long as you can. Eventually, like almost all of your fellow dieters, you fall off the wagon. Life just isn't worth living without an occasional piece of birthday cake. Dieting doesn't make your life longer; it just makes it seem longer. So, like your neighbors, you yo-yo your life away. And, I repeat, it is medically established that each time you discipline yourself to the hunger of your diet, then finally go off your diet, it is harder to lose weight on your next diet. This is a no-brainer. The pattern of hunger teaches your metabolism to hang on to food. Your metabolism learns to work ever more efficiently until it becomes almost impossible to lose weight no matter how little you eat.

All right then, big deal! Being hungry makes your body hang on to weight, so being full obviously makes it ever easier for your body to lose weight. Logically, obviously, scientifically, the converse of a fact leads to the result opposite of that fact.

The equations are simple:

**DEPRIVATION, DIETING — EVER HARDER TO LOSE WEIGHT**
**REPLETION, FULLNESS — EVER EASIER TO LOSE WEIGHT**

There is just one problem. This simply can't be true. There is a limitless list of diets based on deprivation and hunger. There have to be some diets based on the converse. I am not a nut. Since all the doctors of nutrition in their white coats spend all their days in the lab and none has come up with this converse, that fullness makes you lose weight, this converse must be wrong!

There is one difficulty with this thesis. The white coated nutritional PhDs have failed to produce a single diet that works for any length of time. The cemetery is full of their failures.

It is hard to accept hopelessness. Everyone I talk to feels that many diets have failed, but, certainly, some have succeeded. After all, dieting is a scientific challenge, and science always, eventually, comes up with an answer. The obesity all about us is growing till now nutritionists call it "globesity." A prominent doctor said that when medical leaders and nutritionists gather and the subject comes up of the ever increasing globesity and the doom in store for humanity, these authorities just throw up their hands in despair.

At one seminar a nutrition expert said to me, "I keep thinking of *On the Beach*." Nevil Shute wrote about a nuclear war in the Northern Hemisphere. The radioactive fallout was carried by wind currents to the Southern Hemisphere. The fallout killed a few people and then started to kill whole populations. People around the world heard of the fallout and felt sorry for the victims, but they knew that the problem would be solved very soon — long before it poisoned their own country and their own neighborhoods. Science had solved one problem after another; the fallout was just another problem that science would surely solve.

The fallout kept spreading until all of humanity was poisoned. The last people to be hit by the fumes were the Australians. Nevil Shute dwells on the confidence these last survivors felt in the power of science to solve scientific challenges. Until the last minute, just before the fallout hit them, people were sure that science would come to the rescue. The government had issued poison pills to make death quick and easy. As the last humans took their pills they were still in shock and disbelief that science could fail them.

This "*On the Beach*" syndrome is accurate. When I discuss the fact that all diets have failed, I meet with the same blank stare that I must be wrong. Oh yes, many diets have failed, but surely some of them must have succeeded. Weight control is a scientific question: science will surely give us the answer. But will it? So far science has failed to create a diet that works, and time is running out.

My sisters and I have spent hours evaluating the two decades of work that led us to our fullness program. It is so simple that we should have developed it in no time at all. What's the big deal? Study the new foods as they come on the market and pick the ones that are so low in calories that you lose weight while being full. The fact that it took three of us decades of intensive effort tells us that there was a lot more to the process than just choosing foods. There were menacing roadblocks that we had to push aside.

THE FIRST ROADBLOCK was the validity of seeking slenderness. It is true that in those days there was no UN pronouncement about the horrors of globesity. Nevertheless there were strong indications that excess weight was destructive to everything from the heart to the ankles. There should have been wholehearted approval of our efforts to create our fullness program. There was no such approval.

I've presented you a program that is simple and delightful. Eat the new foods as I have described them and you will be full and slender. I wish that the process of developing this program had been simple and delightful. It wasn't. The development of this program was painful. The idea for this program began to grow twenty-some years ago. The first indications of globesity were appearing. On the other hand there were a multitude of diets and diet foods flooding the market. The very number of the diets began to puzzle me. They all used a single format. Cambridge and Powter and Simmons, Phil, etc. all had formulas which would lead you to slenderness. The guts of their programs were all the same. Testimonial followed testimonial showing the size 3X man or woman pronouncing that they had been obese before they went on the diet and now they were perfect slenderellas. The huge "before" pants and the slender "after" pants were the standard props.

The very number of these diets began to puzzle me. Then I read Jane Brody's comment that the very number of these diets proved that none of them worked. If any one of them had worked there would be no need for the others. Meanwhile, she said, diet experts and publishers were making out very well on the new diets which they promised to be absolutely effective. Each had testimonials galore which featured before and after pictures to prove that this diet would turn you from size sixteen to size six.

I subscribed to these promises till I was in my thirties. It took all my courage to grasp the truth of Jane Brody's statement that these diets were failures. Even more wrenching to my emotions was the corollary that the ads and the testimonials were invalid. As a normal American woman I assumed that advertising puffed its products and exaggerated their merits. Still, it was almost impossible for me to grasp Jane Brody's statement that none of these diets worked and therefore the tests and testimonials were invalid. To this day I find it hard to grasp the obvious fact that, if any one of the diets worked or if any of the testimonials were valid, that diet would take over the market and make everyone slender today. It may be a reflection on my immaturity that I still can't come to terms with this obvious fact. I know that everyone who goes on a diet loses weight at first and then regains it in the yo-yo syndrome. I have been in the field for years. I have read the authorities who announce clearly that there is no diet that is effective for any length of time. Still, if you woke me in the middle of the night and asked me, "Are all the diets failures and are all the testimonials invalid?" I would probably say that there has to be some diet that works and that there had to be some testimonial that was valid.

---

My sisters and I have tried to figure out what makes us unique. We don't have a lot of the technical expertise that a lot of the experts boast. We do, however, have one awareness that none of them seem to grasp. Our approach is uniquely effective because we start with the assumption of the omnipotence of hunger as fundamental to all life on earth. The other 300 diet authors gloss over the ravenous, irresistible force of this primal drive. Freudians argue that the sex drive is the primary human drive. I don't see how the two drives can be separated. These drives are the two essentials to life.

The first one-celled protozoa were mouths and stomachs. Their sole activity was to seek food and to try to avoid being food for someone else. Each step of the development of life is simply a higher level of seeking food and postponing the time of being food for the predator higher on the food chain. Now, a billion years later, the deer grazes all day and runs to escape being food for the wolf; the lion sleeps 18 hours a day to gather energy for his sprint to kill the deer and eat it before the lion starves. Many lions die of starvation. Almost all humans labored from dawn to dusk in rice paddies or wheat fields. With luck they gathered enough nourishment to be able to get up and work in the fields the next day. Life is hunger; hunger is life. It may be that a time will come when hunger is not the single driving force in human life, but that time is in the far distant future. Until recently, in most societies, the full rounded belly was the sign of prosperity and it was the skinny beggar who was the outcast. In Muslim countries the sheik filled his harem with the fattest possible maidens. A virgin's price went up in direct proportion to her poundage. A good mother's job was to keep her nubile daughter as motionless as possible so that she wouldn't lose fat by moving, and to cram her with food from morning until night.

<hr/>

Through the ages, wealth was used primarily to buy exotic foods. In the Middle Ages spices were worth more than gold. Magellan lost all but one of his ships on his trip around the world. The pepper and cloves and other spices that were brought back in this single ship brought a profit many times the cost of the whole original fleet. The search for the "Spice Islands" was the force behind the discovery of the New World.

The most brilliant court in Europe was the French court of Louis XIV. His chefs concocted lavish dishes for the Sun King and his huge court. We still have recipes from that era. After giving the ingredients of meat, spices, vegetables etc. the final step was usually to add "one liter of attar of roses" (perfume) — to kill the stench of the unrefrigerated game.

Our founding fathers left detailed records of their cuisine. They were not particularly big men — George Washington at 6'1" was something of a giant. The amounts they consumed were staggering. Breakfast for a tradesman, not a workingman but a tradesman, was a chicken, a dozen eggs, a dozen biscuits, etc. Any good trencherman would wash this down with a half-dozen bottles of wine, ale or cider. We know the size of their bottles; we have many in museums. We have some idea of where all this ended up in Benjamin Franklin's suggestion of awards for creative contributions to humanity. Both Franklin and Twain wrote many risqué essays. In one of them Ben Franklin suggested that the highest award should be given to the man who created the greatest boon to mankind — an elixir that would turn flatulence (gas) into perfume.

This passion for food is evident when Faust sold his soul to the devil and was asked what he'd want in return. His wish was for a bunch of grapes, even though it was wintertime. It would be easy to fill pages about the excesses of the wealthy in the search for taste novelties. The Roman banquet hall was built around a marble vomitorium. After gorging, the reveler put a feather down his throat and, after vomiting, started eating all over again. The Rajahs in India were served monkeys whose heads were clamped tight so that the animals could not move while the diners ate the brains of the living creatures. The wealthy Chinese maxim paralleled an old French saying. "The only diversion equal in importance to eating is talking about food."

This monomaniacal absorption with food was bad enough in ancient days when it had its basis in reality. Famine beset every society. In time of famine, there was no canned food or frozen food to fall back on. In time of famine people ate rats, twigs, and even their own children. Most American families have traditions of famine. The Irish family recalls the great grandfather whose children starved to death in the potato famine. Jewish children learn about the starvation in the Old Country. Every American child who leaves food on his plate is lectured about the "starving children in India or Africa."

I don't believe that any of the nutrition experts gives proper importance to the inexorable power of this primal drive. One after another offers a food plan that prescribes "add a teaspoon of finely chopped chives to the olive oil and marinate 6 ounces of scrod for 20 minutes." After you finish your tiny dinner YOU SIMPLY STOP. Richard Simmons sold millions of his "Deal-A-Meal." You ate your broiled scrod and then "stopped." The Duchess of York, speaking for Weight Watchers, announces her variation of the same theme. She gives you so many ounces of broiled scrod to eat and then tells you to "stop." All the medical authorities agree that diets work for a short time and then fail miserably. One cannot overcome the irresistible power of the hunger mechanism with verbalization of a four-letter word "stop."

---

I am convinced that none of these nutrition "experts" have studied the history of food. The hundreds of millions of years of endless hunger is a tsunami, an irresistible tidal wave that washes out one novelty diet after another. We see the futility of trying to fight this tidal wave. Ever more articles and diet books are being churned out. Atkins sold 15 million copies of his "diet books." The result is ever more obesity. At his death Atkins was described as "grossly obese."

The time may come when the plenitude of food becomes imprinted in the human psyche. Till that day any diet based on hunger is doomed to failure. The memory of hunger is irresistibly strong. This memory dooms diets based on deprivation and hunger to fail miserably, as they do. Only a fullness program, which fulfills this hunger drive, can bring lasting slenderness.

There have been about three hundred published diets in the last century. Aside from the diet books there are innumerable radio and television programs devoted to dieting. It is no exaggeration to say that almost every one of the scores of women's magazines features an article on weight loss practically every issue. These total tens of thousands of articles on weight loss. The primary theme is always the same. Resist your hunger drive. Strengthen your character. Learn to live with less nourishment — with hunger.

Everyone knows the classical programs of weight loss:

Optifast (Now varied as Medifast), limit yourself to a shake for at least one or two meals a day. DEPRIVATION—HUNGER.

The Hollywood Diet — another liquid diet plan like Optifast. These were popular a few years ago. I know tons of people who tried this diet. They lost a lot of weight at first. Practically all ended up regaining the lost weight, and then some. DEPRIVATION—HUNGER.

Slim·Fast. Drink two cans of liquid a day and have a sensible meal. This giant program won tens of millions of adherents. I loved the idea and tried it. When I couldn't stay on this regimen because I didn't find the shakes filling enough, I created my own shake. People must agree with me that the Slim·Fast shake is inadequate because Slim·Fast has taken a catastrophic dip in sales. Its program: DEPRIVATION—HUNGER.

Pritikin forbids processed food such as white bread and eggs and most types of fat. The dieter lives on whole grains, fruits and vegetables. DEPRIVATION—HUNGER.

Ornish's Lifestyle Diet. This strictest of diets limits one to 10 percent fat, no fish, nuts or chicken. It is even more limiting than Pritikin. DEPRIVATION—HUNGER.

Richard Simmons provided his followers with cards listing foods and their calories. His "Deal a Meal" was simply a calorie count with the command "just stop."

DEPRIVATION—HUNGER.

Weight Watchers changed the name of "Deal A Meal" to the Points system. The Duchess of York repeats the same message. "Eat the number of points we assign you and then stop." DEPRIVATION—HUNGER.

The Zone Diet is a complicated program of mathematics. At each meal you have to calculate an intake of 40 percent carbohydrates, 30 percent protein and 30 percent fat. The basic message is still limitation of intake. DEPRIVATION—HUNGER.

The hottest diet of recent times, by far, is Atkins with his low carb religion. Everyone loses weight on Atkins. A good part of the loss is due to the cut in caloric intake. How much cheese and bacon can one eat in a day? What is life without a piece of birthday cake or a cocktail? I know many people who started on Atkins, but I don't know anyone who could stay on it indefinitely. As you came out of it you put back all the weight plus extra pounds for good measure. The diet is based on ketosis — a shock to the system when the fat and protein eaten replace almost all the carbohydrates. Once you modify the system and start eating more carbohydrates, you are out of ketosis. This diet deprives you of the nourishment that is at the basis of the food pyramid, the breads, vegetables etc. The long-range health problems loom menacingly. Atkins claimed to be on his diet all his life; he was a poster boy for his own teaching. At his death, his detractors said he was "grossly obese," his supporters said he was merely "obese." In any event his basic teaching was DEPRIVATION—HUNGER.

It would be repetitive and boring to recount the scores of other diets that have streaked over the horizon and then disappeared. They all have several factors in common. They all demand that the dieter limit either the amount or the kinds of foods he eats. They call the dieter to account. He must have the self-discipline to follow the regimen or he must feel the guilt of being a moral failure. They all assume that to follow one's natural desires leads to disaster. Finally, none of them takes full advantage of the marvelous new foods that are tasty, filling, low in calories and readily available.

I was stunned long ago when I first read Jane Brody's statement that none of the current diets are working. Jane Brody is the nutritional columnist for the *New York Times*, the most prestigious newspaper in the world. She has been the authority in the field for almost half a century. Her statement came as a thunderclap to me when I first read it. Since no diets are working, and humanity is becoming more and more obese, the inevitable result will be four hundred pound teenagers. I read her statement as a pronouncement of doom to the human species, a science fiction-type prediction marking the end of the world.

I read her pronouncement with a combination of horror and yet of selfish relief. I had heard such prophecies in the past. I knew in theory that everything looks hopeless. But seeing the statement in print and knowing that this judgment is offered by a top authority made it earthshaking to me. Tragically, time has proven her right.

I don't like being a prophet of doom. I also find that I am unpopular with some of my friends when we discuss the future of globesity. It seems unthinkable that globesity is running rampant — out of control. We see pieces of the epidemic covered on the news and in the news magazines. Even though we can see the pieces that make up the future of doom, when it comes to putting the pieces together, we balk. We can't envision a world of 400-pound teenagers and 500 pound adults.

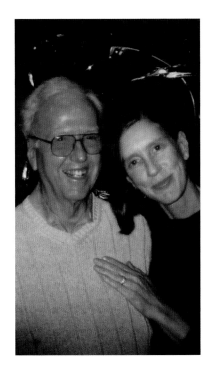

We are the Australians of "On the Beach." We see all the pieces, but we shy away from putting the pieces together. The human can't face the prospect of doom.

There is a story of a soldier who went to a fortuneteller. He said, "My battalion is going to attack the enemy at dawn. What do you foresee will happen? "The fortune teller said, "All but one of the 1000 men in your battalion will be killed." The soldier gasped, "Oh, my poor buddies."

What is happening can't happen. We might be destroyed in nuclear warfare or by pollution or deadly epidemics of viruses. Surely it is preposterous to think that we can be destroyed simply because we can't stop eating.

The graphs are inexorable. They point to an ever-intensifying globesity that will destroy us. The limiting factors are gone. We described previously how the farmer had to be lean for two reasons. He spent the day behind the plow, so he couldn't function if he were obese. He had to be on guard against human and animal predators and he had to be ready for battle when the lord of the manor called him. He had to be slender to function and to live. Only the wealthy and the aristocrats could afford to be fat because they didn't need physical labor to live and they had guards to protect them. They could afford to be fat, so they were fat. Now we are all aristocrats. We don't have to work physically to earn our livings. We have police and soldiers to protect us. We can afford to be fat, so we are fat.

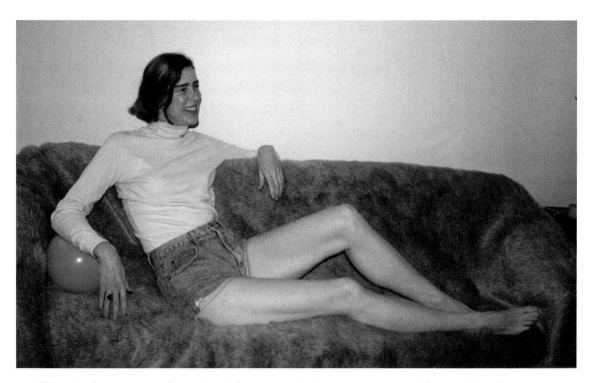

We don't want to face the bitter truth, but we cannot live a lie. Our present programs are leading to ever-greater obesity and to doom.

On the other hand this prophecy of doom made us feel that our theories must be right. Since all other diets underline the need for deprivation — hunger, and since none of them works, it certainly indicates that it is time for a revolutionary new approach to the whole problem. Each diet book follows the same approach as the ones before it. Use your willpower to withstand hunger. This method has never worked but each new book follows the same motif. I heard a story of three gold miners digging for ore. Two overturned new earth looking for nuggets. The third followed behind the other two and dug where they had previously turned the soil. They accosted him and said, "What are you doing? You know there's no gold there. "His response was "Yes, but the digging is so much easier here." The sheer number of these diets indicates that I am right. Since these hundreds of diets are all based on enforcing hunger in the dieter, and since they have all failed, then, surely, the hunger approach must be wrong.

Human nature requires that we need hope in order to survive. When I talk to my friends about the history of diets they all agree that many have failed, but they are sure that "some of them have worked."

I often quote my mother who remembers that in her childhood there were new miracle cures for tuberculosis in the magazines every week. As long as there were numbers of cures, you know that there was no cure. Once streptomycin was invented, tuberculosis ceased to be an unsolvable problem, and the articles on new cures stopped appearing, because the problem was solved. It boggles my mind too, that none of the hundreds of diets has worked, but they haven't. Fighting the hunger drive is fruitless. What if the thousands of soldiers were marching to the wrong beat? What if Johnny was marching to the true beat?

Blaise Pascal was a French mathematician and philosopher. He taught that the sun goes around the earth. When his colleagues reproached him they said, "As a scientist you know that the earth goes around the sun." His response was that he did know that the earth goes around the sun but that he, Pascal, wanted to go to heaven. He explained that even though the Catholic Church might not give him entry into heaven, no one else even offered him entry to heaven, so he said he would continue to teach the church's doctrine that the sun goes around the earth.

———&deg;&deg;&deg;———

We know that none of the hunger — deprivation diets work. I feel that I must be right in striking out in an opposite direction, a diet that has worked for years for my friends and me.

The American still eats from pressure, not from desire. Compulsive eating is on the increase. Obesity is increasingly becoming a national disaster. The fashions this year show no fitted garments. New clothes are shapeless tents to hide the rolls of lard. Losing weight is becoming a major industry. Weight Watchers is one of the growth businesses. Still, the general obesity increases and the alarming spread of gross fatness and diabetes is most obvious in the children and teenagers. A recent study attributes at least 50% of increased teenage disease to increased obesity.

I watched dear friends painfully lose and painfully regain tons of weight. Dieting is the universal punishment for living. Diets are more than useless; they are pernicious. My friends lose weight on a diet, and then regain more weight than they lost, after the diet fails. They end up fatter than ever. One of my friends said facetiously, "If there is a good God in the heaven, he would let me eat all day and still lose weight." Light dawned. I remembered my great-uncle's experience in quitting smoking, when he ate all day and still lost weight. It confirmed in me the conviction that successful weight control depends on cutting out the continual hunger craving.

All the present diets are based on *denying* the basic hunger innate in the human. All these diets *must fail*. Even the Atkins type of diet, which limits the variety of foods that can be consumed, must fail.

The liquid diet is perfect in theory. Imagine eating three delicious "milk shakes" a day as the bulk of your diet. In theory it sounds wonderful. Thick, delicious "shakes" full of crushed ice and strawberry or vanilla or chocolate flavoring. In addition, the powder is full of minerals and vitamins. Soon the whole world would be "California slim." One English woman had the dentist wire her upper teeth to her lower teeth so that she could not open her mouth and, of course, she could not eat. Imagine how desperate she was to lose weight. The dentist left one little aperture between her teeth, just large enough for a straw. This woman planned to live on the liquid shake diet till her fat melted away. Of course, she had to have the wires removed. No one can live on a single kind of food, no matter how delicious. The "shake" type of powder is a superb adjunct to my diet or to any other diet. In itself, though, it is doomed to failure.

The primordial hunger is so great that the human must eat continuously, and must eat every kind of food, continually. Only a program offering an infinitely varied diet can satisfy the human's basic need. The human cannot stand long-term limitations on tastes and texture of food. Any limitation must eventually fail. Once the problem was defined, the answer was self-evident. Eat all day long, of a huge variety of foods, and Nature will give you the perfect body you were meant to have. Thank Heaven the new foods developed over the past few decades enable us to do just that.

No previous diet has been, or could be, successful. Nothing can fight the built-in hunger except this program. The amoeba spends all its time eating and evacuating. The human is no different; it is a long tube with a mouth at one end and a rectum at the other. Its whole built-in mechanism is to eat, search for more food, prepare the food and then eat again. This is the fact that has to be drummed into the participant. You must consciously preoccupy yourself with food more than a dozen times each day. You must put something in your mouth every hour or two.

Our society has made it improper for us to think of food constantly. The proper person represses desire for food. Scarlett O'Hara had to eat a full meal before going to the barbecue, because a southern belle only picks at her food in public. She is never seen to eat. Social pressure tells us that continual preoccupation with food is boorish. Modern man drives his desire for food into the unconscious where it lurks like a time bomb. It explodes and forces him to "pig out." At the same time, the hunger pangs signal the body to go into its famine mode. During periods of starvation the body hangs on to every crumb. Thus fatness and hunger are married; famine and obesity hold hands.

It is precisely this hunger mechanism that we must kill. The body must be relieved of its starvation alarm. You, however, have been programmed to hide your constant hunger. You feel proud when you "don't think of food" for a period of time. You are ashamed of this continual oral preoccupation. You hide from the fact that you're constantly waiting to put something else in your mouth. Sexual researchers have shown that you have a sexual thought every few seconds. Your thoughts about food are equally pervasive.

Reversing this social pressure is the secret of successful slimming. You must associate with people who, like you, have the courage to see that grazing is the basic activity of the human. You must learn, with them, to bring to consciousness this normal, universal, timeless preoccupation with putting something in your mouth. Once you feel the normality of grazing all day of putting something in your mouth every hour or two — you will begin to judo the starvation mechanism. You will replace it with the repletion mechanism. Your body will evacuate food instead of holding it. This is the vital step toward achieving a permanently beautiful body.


A SECOND STUMBLING BLOCK to our acceptance of my program was social tradition. Festive meals and fullness are just not "nice." I studied the nature program's presentation of the bear's year cycle. The bear eats ravenously. When there is plenty of food in the warm months he is slender. When his metabolism switches to the hunger mode of winter the calories he had evacuated now turn to fat. The logic is irrefutable. The awareness of plenty through the feeling of fullness leads to slenderness. The feeling of hunger leads to fat. Our social image, however, of fullness is that of the Roman orgy with Nero at the vomitorium and Henry VIII eating a leg of lamb with the gravy dripping over his enormous paunch. Gentility is summarized in Scarlett's story of the barbecue. A proper young lady doesn't eat — especially in public. A true debutante just picks at her food.

Rena and I had lunch with another business associate just recently. I ate my normal lunch. After Rena and I left the restaurant I pulled out one of my favorite eight-ounce double chocolate muffins and started to eat it. Rena asked why I hadn't chosen a similar muffin that was offered on the dessert tray at the restaurant. I realized, to my dismay that I am still reticent about letting people see how much I eat. Social custom is so strong, that even I find it difficult to exhibit publicly the humongous amount of food that I eat and the Festive meals that keep me slender.

Let me continue my tale of woe. The delightful program, which I presented to you so casually, had yet another hurdle to overcome. Many of the new foods are unknown to much of the public and unknown foods are almost anathema. There is a vivid dislike of the unknown. My sisters and I experimented with the new foods over a period of two decades. We adjusted to them slowly so there was no shock of novelty that confronted us. When we presented strange foods to our friends they often recoiled. We were puzzled that these intelligent, literate friends who were eager to lose weight and who saw that the new foods were composed of super-healthful ingredients still recoiled at making them part of their own lifestyles. In retrospect we see that logic has little to do with emotion. We examined our own prejudices. We know that dog meat is eaten by much more of the human populace than eat beef. We know that Asian doctors and other health authorities rely on dog meat as a basic source of protein and that beef is foreign to them. Yet, we perfectly logical intelligent nutritionists cannot bring ourselves to eat dog meat. Dog meat and guinea pigs and crocodile meat are exotic foods. Much closer to home is ostrich meat and especially buffalo meat. I read the nutritionals on buffalo meat years ago and they are completely positive. Buffalo, and especially beefalo, are superior nutritionally to regular beef. I know this intellectually and I have packages of buffalo meat in my freezer and they have remained in my freezer for months. We who preach intelligent diet are still unconsciously prejudiced against the unknown, the new foods.

It is not only the new foods but the new connotations that cause difficulty. Rena Northrop has been my sister since the beginning. She knows as much about the program as I do. Yet, when I wanted to make my special bagel and my special cream cheese part of a Festive breakfast she hesitated. This combination had been one of her favorite splurges over the years — always resulting in weight gain. Svelte, sexy Rena remembers the time that she weighed 192 pounds. She knows very well that my bagel is 150 calories instead of 400 and that my cream cheese is 35 instead of 200. Still, her conditioning overrode her intellect and she recoiled at the mere words "bagels and cream cheese." My next-door neighbor is a respected young oncologist. She was delighted with our concept and our foods. She objected, however, to our use of the word Festive. When she wrestled with her weight over the years her undoing was always giving in to a Festive binge. She knows very well that we are trying to emphasize fullness but it was hard for her to get past her conditioning about the word "Festive."

There is some excuse for not eating grubs like the South American Indians or for a Jew with a kosher background recoiling at pork. I find it hard though to justify my own difficulty with a wonder food that I recommend as a basic part of our fullness program. The Shirataki noodle is a gift from the heavens. It is made of perfect components such as the yam flour, which is derived from the konnyaku root. Bread is the staff of life for the Western world and we were thrilled to find light bread that is half the calories of the standard product. Pasta is almost as much a staple of our diet as is bread. Here the new noodle is not half the calories of the standard product — it is less than one-fifth the calories. It was almost too good to be true. Here is a healthful noodle that makes pasta no longer a forbidden food but a marvelous aid in slimming down. The catch was that the Shirataki noodle has a slightly springy texture and isn't exactly the pasta that Mother made for me. It is absolutely nutritious and healthful and filling and ridiculously low calorically. Still, the first few times I ate it I felt that I was not eating pasta. This means, of course, that I was not eating Mother's pasta. The standard pasta is limp. Aficionados of pasta want the pasta to be al dente —

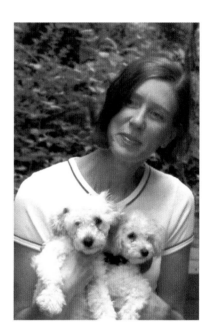

*Dolly & Tutu*

slightly springy. The springiness also makes it more filling for a longer period of time because it takes longer to digest. Still, with all these marvelous qualities going for it, it took me several luncheons of the Shirataki noodle to adjust to this mouth feel. Since it was not the mouth feel Mother had cooked for me it seemed strange and wrong. By now, of course, I have grown to feel that the Shirataki is the right consistency for pasta and that limp, pasty dish Mother prepared is far less interesting. Yes, I have now made the Shirataki my basic pasta. The fact that it took me a few lunches to adjust to this marvelous new food shows again how hard it is for logic to overcome family tradition. The only good foods are the ones Mother made. New taste experiences have to overcome the deep-seated conditioning that they are bad because they are different from Mother's. Even standard foods are suspect when they are not the ones Mother fed us. New forms of familiar foods such as fat-free mayonnaise and cream cheese are suspect.

It took Rena, Eve and me over a decade to overcome our conditioning. Once you know that this conditioning has been confronted and reversed it is much easier to reverse it in your own life. You know intellectually that all the ingredients of our new wonder foods are healthful and doctor-approved. You know that they are low in calories and thus must result in weight loss. Now use our experience to speed your orientation. Know that Rena, Eve and I and dozens of our friends have lived on these foods for years and have become full and slender as a result. If you are conditioned to feel that the new foods have to be suspect because they have so few calories, know that your conditioning is wrong and can be reversed. A diet rich in sweet, sinfully delicious food can lead to healthful slenderness. We in our own lives have reversed the old conditioning. All you have to do is to follow us. Let us not waste any more time. Let us join hands and fill our carts and our pantries with these slenderness-producing new foods.

⸎

A final, and perhaps the most devastating tradition we are breaking with our fullness program is our heritage of Puritan guilt and pain. The Pilgrims gave us our work ethic and tradition of integrity. They also left us a legacy that exalts guilt and pain and looks with horror at laughter and joy and sensuality. In this tradition our fullness program is one that idealizes the sin of gluttony and the weaknesses of vanity and physical repletion. There are still parts of our country that forbid dancing and even baseball on the Sabbath.

The "Lord's Day of Rest" in Puritan society was an occasion for the family to fit into tight shoes and clothing and attend mandatory services. The services lasted as long as seven hours and the two-hour sermon focused on the fire and brimstone that was the fate of anyone who indulged in frivolity and pleasure. Food was the special source of guilt and pain. Talk at meal times had to be limited and only focused on solemn religious themes. During the week the extremity of this sado-masochistic tradition is evident in the lunch period at the farm. The children had been out in the fields at sun-up. When they were called in for lunch they were often made to stand while eating. This extra pain was "good for their souls."

With this background, the whole tenor of our fullness program smacks of gluttony and self-indulgence. With the heritage that exalted fasting and self-denial, it is brutally difficult to look on hunger as evil and satiation as ideal. This tradition has been strengthened by diets that offered cottage cheese and Jell-O for dinner and exalted hunger. We are swimming against the current when we say that it is fullness that triggers the leanness mechanism and that it is the hunger signals that set off fat storage and obesity.

My sisters and I have been wrestling with this tradition in our own lives. To this day I sometimes react against our own fullness program. After a Festive dinner I sometimes run to the scale because the Festive meal smacked of the old "pig out" which resulted in pushing the needle of the scale way up. You, too, must also expect your internal resistance to this reversal of the old dieting principal. You will have to get used to the fact that hunger which used to be promoted as the secret to successful dieting is actually, in truth, the instigator of obesity. Fullness which used to be the no-no is actually the key to slenderness. In due time the validity of these principals will be part of our culture. During the transition period from the old faulty thinking to the new valid thinking, you will have to use your internal fortitude to override your conditioning.

There are two steps to any major scientific development. The first step is the discovery itself. The second step is the time lag in which news of the discovery becomes common knowledge. The first step is ineffective until the second step is completed. The ancients knew that the world was round and that the earth traveled around the sun. This knowledge was wiped out in the Dark Ages and everyone knew that the earth was flat. If you sailed too far, you would fall over the edge. Columbus and Magellan took the chance and now every school child knows that the world is round. Lister showed that there are germs that can be infectious. In some parts of the third world diseases like polio are spreading because the natives won't allow doctors to "stick pins in their women and children." Tomatoes were grown in colonial times because they produced such pretty red fruit. Everyone believed that the fruit was inedible and actually poisonous. A man in Virginia dared to eat a tomato. He found it tasty and nutritious. Immediately the conditioning about eating tomatoes was reversed and everyone ate tomatoes. Incidentally, they erected a statue to this pioneer in the tomato growing area of Virginia.

There was a carnival hustler who had a huge bottle with inch thick glass. He put a snake into the bottle. He bet the customers that they could not keep their hands on the bottle when the snake struck at them. The customers knew very well that no snake-bite could penetrate an inch of solid glass. They put their money down and put their hands on the bottle. Of course when the snake darted at the edge of the bottle, they pulled their hands back and lost their money.

The old fallacies still rule. We still think there are hunger diets that work. New foods that are different from what Mommy served are not real food. There is something morally wrong and anti-God in feeling replete and sexy. My sisters and I have faced these demons and we have overcome them. We are in our fifties or in our eighties and we are slender and full. We have sailed over the edge of the world and we are happy to tell about it. We have eaten the tomato and lived. We have survived injections for preventable diseases and we are the healthier for it. We have kept our hands on the bottle when the snake darted at us and the snake attack was a non-event. We have faced the demons that time would unmask as irrelevant superstition. Don't waste the moments of your life perpetuating the nonsense that hunger leads to slenderness and that the non-Mommy foods are inedible and that God doesn't want you to be satisfied and slender. We have conquered the time lag for you. Come on in, the water is fine. We're enjoying every minute of it. Profit by our experience and join us.

---

I can't emphasize too strongly the stranglehold of guilt on our society. I've studied more than 300 diets in the history of American nutrition. Just as they all limit either the amount or kind of food the dieter must ingest, so do they all stress that discipline and guilt are the forces that make a diet work. It was hard for me to buck their unanimity that guilt is vital for losing weight.

One of the bad experiences of Rena's life was her brief experience with Weight Watchers. She feels that this most popular program is based on sadism and masochism. She had to be weighed publicly, hoping for the cheers of approval if her weight stayed the same or went down. At the same time she would cower inwardly at the anticipation of the stony silence if her weight went up. This public humiliation was a standard routine of the program. How anyone can stand this public humiliation is beyond my comprehension. Private guilt is bad enough; a routine of public humiliation is unbearable to us. It would be foolish, however, to deny the vast and continuing popularity of this program, and it is based on guilt, guilt, and guilt.

It is my understanding that Jean Nadisch founded the Weight Watchers program on the pattern of Alcoholics Anonymous. Here too we have an enormously popular, and very effective weapon against alcoholism. I know of no other "drying out" system as effective and as popular and as enduring. Here again we are faced with the fact that an effective program requires that most powerful of weapons — guilt. I hate to come to this conclusion. I wracked my brain trying to think of some other program that is effective in fighting alcoholism, but I simply couldn't think of any. Antabuse makes drinking unpleasant because its mixture with alcohol makes the imbiber sick, but this is hardly a competitive cure to AA. As with Weight Watchers, I find the process objectionable but there seemed to be no other alternative available.

Guilt is built into the very fabric of our society. "Find out what the children are doing and tell them to stop." Some time ago a national bestseller was "How to be a Jewish Mother." The book opened with a cartoon of the elderly matron standing with her arms crossed. Her facial expression was that of deep hurt. Her message was that she didn't have to tell the children how they have hurt her. Her facial expression was enough. Her children would figure out how they hurt her. Their imaginations would create more guilt in them than any verbal accusations of hers would produce.

This "very funny" theme of creating guilt has become a stock motif in the sitcom and comedy. Who has not seen Doris Roberts destroy her family week after week on "Everybody Loves Raymond"? This weekly program focused around guilt is one of the most watched television programs in the country. Mother announces that creating guilt in the children is her "job." Guilt is the driving force in making the child study and in making the adult succeed. It certainly has been the driving force in every regimen designed to make the dieter lose weight. How then could we hope that our diet can be effective since it is based on fullness? The only guilt, if any, is that one allows hunger pangs to sneak in without being confronted with our gold coin of nibbles. **A diet of fullness is based on gratification and has no room for guilt.**

A parallel with the need for the feeling of guilt is the need for pain. It is axiomatic in our culture that "No pain — no gain." Our national pastimes are watching huge men mash into each other with all the force they can muster. Boxing is even more overt than football. We watch powerful men smash each other's faces and bodies. The movie cowboy works hard all week to earn money for his Saturday night blowout. His one evening of leisure ends in a brawl where furniture is broken and teeth are knocked loose.

There are subtler, but equally insidious evidences of our need for pain. Bill Cosby produced a famous vignette in which he sat on the floor next to the toilet bowl. In the pauses between his drunken vomiting he protested that it was his right to get drunk at the party. He'd worked hard for the time and money and leisure to have this binge. The skit consisted of alternating vomiting and protestations that drunkenness was his rightful privilege.

Even subtler is gambling. Gambling consists of going to a casino and losing money. One can beat a game or several games. No one can beat the house. In the long run you have to lose. The average slot machine takes fifteen or more percent for the house. In six or seven games your money is gone. I was shocked to hear the statistics that the gambling industry makes more profit than all the professional sports, plus the movie industry and music industry COMBINED. Everyone knows that the odds are unbeatable, but millions need the pain of losing through gambling.

Suffering is an end in itself. Diet after diet fulfills this need for hunger, suffering. When the diet fails, and they all have failed, it is the dieter's fault for being weak. After failing with this diet he or she will go on to the next hot new diet, lose weight at first, and then yo-yo.

My program violates our heritage. It looks on hunger and suffering as unnatural and destructive. In the present atmosphere, "If you want to put on ever more weight, keep going on ever more hunger diets." My program of fullness sounds decadent and morally wrong.

I may appear to be immodest, but, I do compare myself to Jocelyn Elders, the Surgeon General of the United States in 1993. One of her grimmest challenges was the poisonous spread of AIDS and other sexually transmitted diseases. Coupled with this contagion was the "illegitimate" birth of almost half the children in the poverty stricken areas. Many of these children are born with AIDS and the other sexually transmitted diseases. My friends and I have worked with these inner city kids. They are by and large lovely youngsters. Most are very unglamorous, desperately poor, with absolutely no positive home life. They are easily seducible by anyone who offers them even the appearance of affection. Because these poor children make the "mistake" of succumbing to someone who offers them what seems to be affection, they must pay the price of nine months of lonely agony. This is followed by at best the loss of the infant to an adoptive family or agency. Otherwise the child must try to provide for the infant, often in an environment of squalor.

These are the rulings of our civilized, advanced society. Dr. Elders offered a program of sex education which included approval of masturbation, which would give the children an outlet for their natural drives with absolutely no down side. Our Puritan background is so deeply entrenched in us that we smashed her and her program and returned to punishment, punishment, punishment and guilt, guilt, guilt.

I resent bombastic diet authorities, especially since almost all of them are, themselves, obese. I bristle when I see tapes of Doctor Atkins chastising poor dieters who have "strayed from his sacred path." I remember my own suffering over the years when I listened to these august teachers espouse their divine wisdom. They were so righteous. Anyone who couldn't stick to their regimen was a sniveling weakling, a fallen soul with no willpower or character. These "authorities" poisoned my teen years. It is still hard for me to accept that diet teachers like Allan North and Dr. Phil, etc. are fatsos. Dr. Thurman has poor little girls send him cash. He sends them body outlines. They are to shade in the parts of the body that his personalized diet will sculpt. He of course is also a pudge. The physical damage these "authorities" have inflicted on kids through their teachings, which result in the yo-yo effect, are hard to imagine. The emotional damage these fat teachers have inflicted on innocent kids is unforgivable. The prime mover to most of these diet authorities is, of course, the almighty buck. There is a lot of money to be made in visiting guilt trips on innocent adolescents. The basic weapon of these snake oil salesmen is the "test." X number of recruits are put on a placebo (a pretend diet). The same number is put on the diet being advertised. After a time both groups are weighed. If there is more weight loss on the group eating the advertised diet, it is obvious that the advertised diet works. Negative results are not reported.

The difficulties of this process are obvious to anyone who knows about experimentation. Even well-meaning doctors unconsciously affect test results. Also, even many reputable tests are fixed. The final truth which makes the rest irrelevant is that there have been tested products supervised by all kinds of authorities. These tests have resulted in huge sales of products and also in huge profits. The end result is that each hot new tested diet soon fades into the background to be replaced by the next hot new tested diet. With all the vaunted tests after tests after tests, which prove how effective they are, each diet has fallen on its face and obesity is worse than ever. These tests tell each fat person that the diet is good and that he or she is the problem. They enhance the guilt of the poor dieter, but they do make tons of money for the snake oil salesmen.

*The New York Times*, January 4, 2004, ran a front page article about the fact that there have never been any real tests as to the effectiveness of any weight loss program. The long article quotes doctors begging the various national weight loss programs to sponsor tests to back up their claims. Of the many national programs none would agree to sponsor a test that was valid in the eyes of the doctors. The only minor exception was Weight Watchers, which did sponsor a real test. The result of the test, however, was most unimpressive. People weighing over 200 pounds lost only about 6.4 pounds after two years. The climax of the article was Dr. Wadden's statement that the modest and temporary weight losses are not a surprise because "no one knows how to elicit permanent weight loss."

The pervasiveness of guilt in sexuality is evident in the laws of our land. In some states a husband and wife can be fined or jailed for having sex with the woman on top. It is easy to laugh at these laws, but they have destroyed untold numbers of lives. Even more than the destruction of life is the guilt that affects even the most sophisticated of us, for our thoughts and feelings. President Carter confessed that he lusted in his heart. He was a born again Christian who accepted Christ as his personal savior. This man, the President of the United States, announced publicly the guilt he carried with him because of a natural sexual desire.

Dr. Elders' positive answer was unacceptable to our culture. Four out of ten Americans consider themselves "born again" and fundamentalist. They are condemning infants to be born with disease rather than find a normal outlet for the natural sexual drives of these inner city children.

In my own area I have been confronted with the same look of disbelief on many in my audience. There is something morally wrong in offering a diet that uses fullness as a means of reaching ideal weight. Will the public accept the diet that rejects guilt and bases its success on positive reinforcement?

# CHAPTER 21

# *Why It Works*

BOO'S ADDRESS AT THE FOOD SCIENCE AND TECHNOLOGY DEPARTMENT OF CORNELL UNIVERSITY, April 29, 2003

### Boo's Patented Festive Cure For Obesity

Dr. Rao, Mr. Cooley, Dr. Padilla, honored guests,

I am grateful for your invitation to present my invention and program. I feel humble in the presence of so many nutritional experts. My own background is not in the sciences; I was a high school English teacher. My interest in nutrition began when I had to face the threat of obesity. Like the rest of my family I tried all the standard diets. As you know they all work for a short time, then they fail. Their promise of weight loss is a misnomer. The standard diet is like a bank account in which you deposit your fat. After awhile you get your deposit back with interest. It was a sobering discovery to see that none of the diets worked. All the vaunted programs and shakes and other weight loss gimmicks are various forms of hype. The testimonials are overt hype. After all the decades and hundreds of diet books and tens of thousands of diet articles *The New York Times* conclusion was simply, "there is, at this time, no proven way of permanent weight loss." The last diet I tried was Slim·Fast, which had a very appealing ad campaign. Drink two delicious shakes a day and eat a sensible dinner. Then you'll be full and slender forever. The thin Slim·Fast shake just didn't do the job for me and I tossed the Slim·Fast diet onto the scrap heap of the other failed diets.

Their ad campaign, though, haunted me. Why couldn't there be two delicious filling shakes a day that could be the basis of a satisfying nutritional program? As I analyzed Slim·Fast I saw that it was as caloric and sugary as the other shakes. It contained little of the ingredients that lead to a feeling of fullness. I couldn't understand the product. The challenge of weight loss is to ingest tasty products, which are as low as possible in calories and as filling as can be. Why they used sugar instead of the new zero calorie sweeteners and why they didn't include more filling ingredients was a puzzle to me. The only reason I could think of was that this was the least expensive way of producing the product.

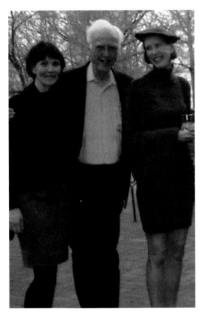

*Celebration Luncheon at Cornell University*

As we began to relate more intimately with the techs and other experts we were constantly confronted with the question of money. The finest sweeteners are expensive. Even more forbidding are the fibers and gums which lead to the sensation of fullness. As we started to use these ingredients the techs warned us that we would price ourselves out of the market. Some of the gums cost fifty cents an ounce. The fat fighters and trace minerals were very pricey. Our response to these warnings about price was that we might have to charge double what the others are charging. This was a chance we were willing to take. It is my belief that a truly slenderizing product would command a market at even two or three dollars a can. The inexpensive product is inexpensive but it just doesn't work. We questioned ourselves as to our judgment. Might the girl in the workforce reject a diet shake that cost her two dollars instead of one? We are counting on the basic wisdom of the American public. Slim·Fast costs less than a Coke. If we could create a product that helped her slender down and costs twice as much she would be wise enough to invest the extra change in the more expensive product for the sake of her health and beauty.

My friends and I had the leisure and determination to undertake this challenge. We felt that we had a chance of producing the kind of shake we had been looking for in Slim·Fast. With ample time on our hands and ample money behind us we felt that we could tap the best brains in the world to produce such a low calorie, delicious, filling shake. If we had known what was in store we might have faltered. We had no idea that it would take more than five years of time and over a half million dollars to make the shake a reality. Over those years we established wonderful relationships with nutritionists and technicians from all over the world. You, Dr. Rao and Herb Cooley and Dr. Padilla know that we were in communication with you at Cornell several times a week over the years. We promised ourselves that if our project succeeded, we would send a portion of the profit to the Nutrition Center at Cornell in honor of your invaluable guidance. I would be remiss if I didn't also mention the support of Patti DeMatteo and Irwin Pearl and thank them publicly for the magnificent equipment they presented to your laboratory on our behalf.

The end result of these labors was the United States patent awarded us in 2002. The patent substantiates the validity of our endeavors. Equally important to us is the response you gave us this morning when we subjected you to our blind taste test. Almost all of you found our shake to be tastier than the three others. It was especially gratifying to hear your comments that our shake made you feel full while the others did not.

You have indulged me in being attentive so far, so I will throw another concept to you. My friends and I began to use our shake as the basis of our filling, tasty, low calorie diet. At the same time we began to find other new products that were produced along our line of thinking. These brand new products use the wonderful sugar substitutes that cut the caloric content drastically. They also use the new fibers, and the new fat substitutes to make their products filling and rich without the caloric and other detrimental aspects of using fat. Now that we have the patent for our shake we are toying with a new project. We plan to launch a formal program of Festive eating. This program is so obvious. Who would not want to eat rich Festive meals and lose weight? We would not only end obesity but we'd offer healthy nutrition that slenders you down while you eat like Henry VIII. We have even toyed with a possible name for our program, "We Have the Cure for Obesity."

You have indulged me so beautifully that I am going to present yet another concept for your consideration. It is the ABC of nutrition that ingesting more calories than we burn leads to weight gain; ingesting fewer calories than we burn leads to weight loss. The problem had always been that low calorie foods were tasteless gerbil food, which could not be sustained as a diet in the long run. Tasty foods were high in calories and led to the obesity epidemic facing us. Finding low calorie food that is the basis of delicious Festive meals solves this problem beautifully. We eat richly while becoming slender.

There is a story of a Southern farmer who was digging in his field to plant cotton. The trouble was that every time he dug into the earth oil spurted out. We were thrilled beyond words with our Festive program, but then we saw a new dividend that seemed to be handed to us. Rena, Eve and I and the others who had worked with us over the years plunged wholeheartedly into the Festive meal program for our own well-being. After we were solidly established at our ideal weight levels we started to confess a secret to each other. Each of us had the experience of overindulging whether it was the extra liquor at a New Years party or the outlandish calories of a delicacy at a special restaurant. Each of us binged and planned to cut back on food to return to our normal weight. The problem that perplexed us was that even after the binges our weight didn't go up. This seemed contrary to the basic law of nutrition. Eat more calories than you burn and the extra calories will be stored as fat.

We are fans of Nova and other nature programs. We watched a series on the bear. The bear has no natural enemies except of course, man. The bear is omnivorous, eating everything from honey to salmon. He eats all day every day. The bear is always at its perfect weight. When food is plentiful he remains lithe and agile to catch his prey. He evacuates excess calories. When the hunger of hibernation approaches he continues to eat with the same frenzy but now the excess calories turn into fat to nourish him over his long winter sleep.

The laws of nutrition don't seem to hold. Eating extra calories in the summer resulted in evacuation. Eating extra calories toward winter resulted in surplus fat. Obviously there is some governing principal that enters the picture beyond just the number of calories. It was our perusal of Dr. Carlton Fredricks and his successors that explained that there is a governing mechanism which keeps the bear at its perfect weight at all times. In times of plenty the bear was at his slenderest for hunting game. In the fall he piled on fat to sustain him in the winter. Put another way, in the summer when he knew there was plenty of food his feeling of fullness set off the mechanism to make him evacuate excess calories. In the hunger of winter his metabolism made him store these calories as fat. The key to his slenderness was his feeling of fullness. This paralleled our own experience. As we became accustomed to the low calorie Festive meals and to feeling full all the time we became the bear in summer. Even when we overate our metabolisms kept us at the ideal weight.

In retrospect we realize that we had always been hungry, the bears in winter. Eve, from her childhood was hammered with the story of the starvation and suffering her family endured over the ages in Europe. Rena's family was raised on stories of the potato famine in Ireland when a third of the population starved to death. I was brought up in a family of the "clean plate club." If I left any morsel to be thrown out I was admonished about the starving children in India and Africa. We all lived in the hunger mechanism. We had all lived as the bears in winter. The hunger mechanism was alerted to turn excess calories into fat. With our new low-calorie Festive meals, we slipped into the mode of plenty. We became the bears in summer. The feeling of fullness based on low calorie Festive meals changed our metabolisms. Even when we exceeded our normal intake our metabolisms kept our weight at its ideal level. This phenomenon will be a subject of research for us in the years to come. We hope to continue to pick the brains of all you doctors and technicians. Perhaps, some time in the future you will invite us back to present our findings on this additional dividend to our low calorie Festive meal program for curing obesity.

I wish I had the poetic ability to express my gratitude to you all for your support and cooperation over the years culminating in this beautiful celebration today. Since I haven't the poetic ability to put into words the beautiful emotions in my heart, let me conclude simply by saying "thank you."

## Briefly, Then, My Program Is

## The OPPOSITE WAY of becoming slender

The present diets have failed. Most of the diet doctors and teachers are themselves pudgy or fat. It is time to take an opposite approach and to succeed. The successful approach is to take the converse of what we are sure about dieting.

Authorities agree:
1. Feeling hungry makes your body hang on to weight.
2. Each time you diet it becomes harder to lose weight on your next diet.
I have based my Fullness Program on the converse of this fact.
**Just as feeling hungry makes your body hang on to weight, feeling full makes your body shed weight.**
(The natural world is full of examples of this principle)

To establish the feeling of fullness you could eat rich foods with the resulting weight gain, or you can achieve the same feeling of fullness with my program based on low-calorie, FILLING foods that also give you the feeling of fullness without weight gain. Once the feeling of fullness is established, your body will evacuate excess weight.

# CHAPTER 22

# The Awful Truth About Obesity

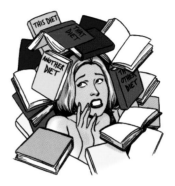

MY BOOK HAS BEEN MANY YEARS IN THE MAKING. I have exposed its premises to more than 3,000 readers. The ones who grasped its ideas and lost the weight understood the premises on which it is based. Those who didn't grasp these concepts did not follow our program and did not lose weight. Here are the two premises:

One: Obesity is the single greatest threat to the health of humankind. It is horrendous now, and it is increasing at an alarming rate. This is common knowledge. Unfortunately, many of my readers trivialize this fact. Sure, obesity is bad, but so are malaria, AIDS, cancer, and juvenile delinquency. We have lived with these other problems, and now we will live with the problem of obesity.

There are telltale signs of this trivialization of the horrors of obesity. These readers ignore the fact that injection needles have had to be made longer because of the increased fat tissue in modern youth, or that autopsies on five-year-olds killed in accidents show blocked arteries. Evidence of this trivialization is a comment such as "I can tell the difference between Classic Coke and Diet Coke." This obese person will consume 17 teaspoons of sugar per drink because of a fancied taste preference. This is as insane as the remark of a tuberculosis victim who says he won't take streptomycin, because the capsules are a shade of blue that he doesn't like. Recognizing the severity of the obesity epidemic is necessary in order for you to benefit from my fullness program.

Two: My fullness program is based on the principle of repletion. Previous diets have been based on the exact opposite — hunger. They limit the amount and/or the kind of food the dieter can consume. Authorities agree that all the old diets have failed. They point to the fact that obesity is continually on the increase. If any of the old diets had worked, there would be a dip on the chart of the growth of obesity. The failure of the old diets indicates the need for a change in direction. Instead of deprivation diets, it is time to turn to my fullness program.

Many of those on whom I tested my theories could not shake their conviction that there are deprivation diets that are succeeding, and so a change in direction is unnecessary. The 60 years of heavy advertising about the amazing results of the Cambridge, Grapefruit, Hollywood, Atkins, Slim·Fast, Weight Watchers diets, etc., have brainwashed many Americans. Surely those thousands of before-and-after ads must have some validity! Surely the $50 billion a year spent on the diet industry cannot be all failure and fraud.

The sad fact is that all the previous diets are failures. If any one of them had worked, the obesity indicators wouldn't keep rising, and there wouldn't be the need for a radical new approach such as my fullness program.

"My mind is made up; don't confuse me with the facts!" The tragic fact announced by our government, the United Nations, and the major diet authorities is that deprivation diets of the past have all failed, and that a new approach is needed. If you cannot come to terms with this awful truth, you will lack the motivation to follow my fullness program and benefit from it.

# CHAPTER 23

# The Urgency of My Program

OBESITY HAS BECOME A PLAGUE affecting young and old around the world. There is no cure for the plague in the present. The more remedies for obesity that are being offered, the more obesity spreads. A prominent doctor said, "When the experts talk about the future they simply throw up their hands."

The bewilderment concerning this plague is understandable. Its elements are foreign to human experience. Throughout history humans have lived with hunger as the threat, and slenderness as automatic. There was always a famine or drought in the offing. Slenderness was built in. Hunting and farming are both marginal means of subsistence. Even the lean hunter or farmer can barely make it. An obese hunter or farmer simply couldn't survive.

This equation was constant. Hunger was the challenge to be met; slenderness was a given. It is in the very recent past that the whole situation has turned upside down. Labor has become a small part of work. In the U.S., until the 1930's, most people lived on farms. Machinery did only a small fraction of heavy labor. Now Americans are city dwellers and machinery does the labor. Our work now consists of pushing a mouse, and obesity is no hindrance to survival. Even walking is a lost art. Since we can survive without manual work, and since the army and the police protect us from attack, we no longer have to be slender to survive. For the first time in history we can be safe, make a living, and be fat.

The only similarity to our condition in olden days was the situation of the noble and the wealthy. They, too, had no need to labor physically and had guards to protect them. Without the need for leanness for survival, they became obese. Nero, Henry VIII, the Titian and Reubenesque women were all forerunners of our present "privileged fat society."

Another constant through the ages was the emotional involvement with food. A major part of each day was devoted to procuring food or preparing food. Even this emotional involvement with food is now gone. Only a hobbyist makes bread anymore. When food required attention, the diner was emotionally ready for repletion by the time he sat down to eat. When the stomach was full he was ready to quit.

The emotional force behind hunger and repletion is neglected in nutritional thinking today. The experts teach of calories, not of feelings. The truth is that in all aspects of life emotions are primary in shaping us for the good or for the bad. Feeling unfulfilled leads to gluttony. Feeling full leads to satiation. The Whopper has more calories than many a French gourmet dish. Ordering it and finishing it in minutes leads to gluttony. Dining slowly on coq au vin, which is simply a piece of chicken, leads to satiation. The emotions are powerful in conditioning us. It takes at least 20 minutes for the brain to register that ingestion has begun. In our day the diner has finished his Whopper long before the 20 minutes are up and thinks longingly of more food even before he leaves the lunchroom.

The French are a culture which has so far maintained this emotional absorption with food. "The only thing as important as eating is talking about food." They dine leisurely on sauces rich with cream and egg yolks. Focused on food as they are, they stop eating when the stomach is full. They therefore eat far fewer calories than we do, with far less diabetes and heart disease etc. from obesity. In our culture food, like other pleasures, has always been an enemy. The cure for obesity is to stop thinking of food, and certainly to cut down on eating food. This is still the prevalent outlook. Suffer, be hungry, and your obesity may go away.

Every diet but mine is a form of hunger. Richard Simmons — "Deal a Meal" says "Eat and then stop." Weight Watchers — Duchess of York promotes "Deal a Meal" under a different name. Atkins says, "Almost never touch carbohydrates." The spread of these hunger disciplines has resulted in the spread of obesity. It is basic psychology to know that repression of any instinct results in intensification of that instinct. The Victorians put lace tablecloths over piano legs lest they be sexually suggestive. This sexual repression resulted in legalized prostitution for ten year olds. Since the promotion of deprivation increases obesity, the experts are trying to put out the inferno of obesity by prescribing more hunger. They are fighting the fire by pumping gasoline onto the flames. Trying to fight obesity through prescribing more hunger is ludicrous. It is no wonder that, "if you want to gain weight go on a diet." It is no wonder that the more diets offered, the greater the national obesity.

The answer to obesity is to follow a program of fullness, where we approach food as a friend and prepare ourselves emotionally for repletion. The method will be to create personal diets that are tasty, low calorie, and filling. Every one touches on these basic factors. **There is no diet, however, that I know of, until mine, that is based solely on this trinity: frequent food and drink that are 1. tasty, 2. low calorie, and 3. filling.** These foods are at hand. The last 10 years has seen the creation of delicious, low calorie foods that were not even imagined in my mother's day. Select judiciously from these new foods and you will find them to be tasty and filling and easy to use. It takes no great effort to slather 5 calorie margarine on 40 calorie toast with low-calorie jam or cinnamon with no-calorie sweetener. There are many other foods that exist or that are being created based on these three criteria — tasty, low-calorie, and filling. All that's left is for you to make these ideals into realities.

CHAPTER 24

# The Fountain of Life

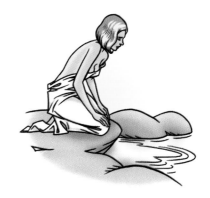

I CANNOT THINK OF THE SUBJECT OF DRINK without recalling a Black History professor of mine who used to talk about Father Divine. Father Divine was born George Baker and in 1915 became an evangelist. Instead of speaking about God and Jesus, he announced that he was the new embodiment of God. He was now the Divine Father and insisted that he be called Father Divine. In the course of time he amassed a huge fortune and married a black woman and a white woman. No one could question God's actions and he was God.

Father Divine attracted tens of thousands of worshippers from among the poorer classes of the urban black communities — especially on the east coast. He renamed his followers with angelic names like Peace, Love, and Serenity. He made them scrupulously honest. They would try to make restitution for any wrong they'd ever done. There are stories of his "Angels" who traveled long distances to pay a store owner a penny for a piece of candy they'd stolen years before. Hiring one of his followers as a domestic was something of a coup. She would be scrupulously honest and conscientious in her work.

God does not function as humans do. Father Divine was open in his relationship with his wives. His followers, though, were subject to a different set of rules. They had to be celibate. Even husbands and wives could have no marital relationships. One of his female worshippers was married to an outsider. The husband demanded his rights as a husband. She appealed to Father Divine. He gave her a framed picture of himself which she took to bed with her every night. She used it as a buffer to prevent her husband's sexual advances.

Father Divine's worshippers turned all their assets and all their daily earnings over

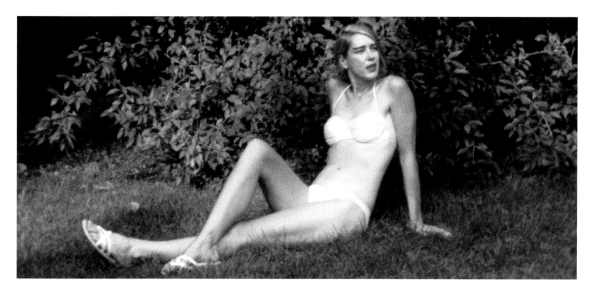

to him. He, in turn, provided them with all their physical needs. He bought various "heavens." One of them was next to the Roosevelt estate on the Hudson. Several were in New York City. These "heavens" provided dormitory-like accommodation — clean cots and washrooms. Most important of all they provided the ultimate in fancy foods — chicken in various forms.

Today chicken is a mass production industry. This mechanization makes poultry by far the cheapest of meats. Before the mechanization chickens ran semi-wild on the farms; they ran off much of their body weight. They were fed by hand, they were slaughtered by hand, and their feathers were plucked by hand. In an A&P advertisement in 1936 roast beef and corned beef sold for 19 cents a pound. Chicken sold for 39 cents a pound. When Herbert Hoover predicted the end of the depression and the coming of prosperity, he promised that if he were re-elected every American would have a car in his garage and a chicken in every pot.

The irresistible attraction of the "heavens" was that chicken was the climax of the evening meal. The worshiper labored hard all day and turned his earnings over to Father Divine, but in the evening there was the ultimate reward of chicken in one of many various forms.

How could Father Divine afford this most expensive of meats for all his followers? One device he used was the lavish dispensation of liquid. Every meal began with a 12-ounce tumbler filled with water. Since Father Divine or one of his representatives blessed the water in his name, the faithful had to drink all of it. This course was followed by a large bowl of soup which also enjoyed Father Divine's blessing. In addition to the water and the soup there were other seasonal drinks like cider or fruit juice which also received the divine blessing. By the time the main course was served the faithful could just pick at the chicken and trimmings. Reluctantly the staff had to clear away the almost untouched chicken, which was saved for use the next day.

My history professor's recounting of this story was pleasant and positive. Obviously there was a con artist element to Father Divine. The fact is, though, that his followers were more slender, healthier, and happier than ever before. Some attribute their superb state of being to the power of Father Divine. I am a cynic and am sure that drinking all that liquid was a real factor in their well-being.

━━━━◦●◦━━━━

An intelligent diet should be part of a wholesome health regimen. Proper food habits must be matched with proper drinking habits. The classic adage is you must drink at least six to eight glasses of water a day. You must "urinate clear."

You are a civilized person or you would not be reading this book. After you bathe, the bath water is quite clear. You would never let yourself get so soiled that the bath water would be dirty. At the same time, you may have no qualms about letting dirt build up inside you. You accept the fact that you are dirty inside if you let your urine become colored. I have been to dinner dances at posh hotels where the powder rooms smelled like abandoned farm outhouses.

Equate your outer cleanliness with inner cleanliness health. The water after you bathe is practically clear; drink enough so that your urine is practically clear. Your outer hygiene will be matched by your inner hygiene.

Esthetics is only part of the reason for drinking at least eight glasses of water (liquids) a day. Drinking water is, in itself, a marvelous boost for slimming.

Your mother may well have followed the Stillman diet some fifty years ago. Dr. Stillman was the Atkins/Pritikin/Tarnower of his day. HIS WHOLE WEIGHT LOSS PROGRAM WAS BASED ON DRINKING ENORMOUS QUANTITIES OF WATER BEFORE, DURING AND AFTER MEALS. His diet was as effective as any other diet has ever been. The "Stillman diet" was a household phrase for years.

The therapeutic value of water has been known through the ages. Wealthy Europeans patronized the "spa" for every conceivable ailment. Many Victorian romances take place in spas. Bath, Ems, Evian and Baden Baden were the gathering places of aristocracy. There they sat in the mineral waters, waded in the mineral waters and, above all, drank the mineral waters.

This practice of "taking the waters" goes back to Greco-Roman days and is even mentioned in Egyptian literature. Certainly, a practice that is so universal and has lasted for so many ages may have value. Since modern medicine can find no therapeutic value in the sulfur and other minerals, the benefit must have been derived simply from drinking large quantities of water.

Yes, water and air are the essentials of life. A human can live several weeks without food, but he dies after only a few days without water. One of the discoveries of the Second World War was the means of getting fresh water for our sailors adrift on the ocean. The sailor adrift on the salt water is the very symbol of irony; water, water, everywhere, but it's all salt. The poor sailor is doomed without fresh water. Over the centuries no one figured out how to save him. Fish are plentiful and their bodies are full of fresh water. Fishing is no problem, but it would take a pressure grinder to squeeze the fresh water out of the fish flesh. It wasn't till modern times that the American Navy devised a method of extracting fresh water from the fish. The sailor had a pressure grinder with him — his teeth. Chewing raw fish may not be delectable but provided fresh water and saved lives.

The plentiful fresh water that we have on tap has made us forget that clean fresh water is the essential for life health and is an endangered resource. This liquid of the Gods has actually fallen into disfavor. Whole industries have grown up to color water and to sugar it. I see inner-city children spend a large part of each day's lunch money on colored sugar water. They have to spend a dollar on Pepsi or Coke because the fast-food place serves no water. Even some of the more expensive restaurants serve water only on request.

Most countries have used human waste to fertilize their crops (night soil). Since they suffered from impure water supplies they had to boil the water that was poisoned by human waste. The boiled water had to be flavored and served as tea or coffee or as wine or beer. Even today we know how disastrous it is to drink the water in countries like Mexico. In our country, we have unlimited drinkable water. We can easily drink the two quarts needed daily to make our urine clear.

Drinking a glass of hot water, flavored with lemon or any other juice upon arising, used to be a staple of the healthy American regimen. This practice should be resumed. Demand a full glass at the restaurant and tip accordingly. Be as clean inside as you are outside. You will be healthy and you will maintain your beautiful body.

The bottom line is that you can get the needed amount of liquid only if you include fresh water. The other forms of liquid have built-in limitations. If you drank eight 8 oz. cups of coffee a day the caffeine would make you jumpy. Tea has plenty of caffeine too. Even decaffeinated coffee is filling, especially with milk and sweetener. It would be just as hard to drink the needed amount of liquid in the form of soft drinks. They are filling in a bad way because of their sugar and carbonation and sodium and coloring. Wine is no answer either. Wine is classified as a food rather than a liquid. One of the old parlor game questions was, "if you were stuck on a desert island, could you live longer on water alone or wine alone." Most people answered, "wine." They figured that wine would fill the need for liquid and also offer nourishment. The fact, though, is that wine has caloric content roughly equal to fish, ounce for ounce.

You can live for weeks without food, but you die in days without water. Wine is a food. Ditto for beer which, on caloric count, is as filling a food as fish. As you open the beer can or drink your white wine on the rocks, picture the fact that you are doing the equivalent of eating a bowl of cereal or a fruit cup. As you drink your tall glass of water, picture yourself at the side of a clear bubbling brook drinking from the fountain of life. The way to get your 48 to 64 ounces of water a day is to drink at least 32 ounces of pure clear water. You can then make up the rest in the form of soda, coffee, etc.

Most of my friends would never serve tap water at dinners and cocktail parties. They serve oceans of Perrier, Evian, etc. I do not serve or drink any of the bottled waters. They are, to me, a fraud. The tests I have studied show that they contain more bacteria and germs than tap water. I do have a filter on my kitchen faucet (there are any number of modestly priced fixtures to attach to your tap). The water that comes out is not only cheaper, but also purer and tastier than the bottled stuff.

Once you establish the pattern of drinking the required amount of water a day, and urinating clear, you will feel repelled at the thought of your past when you had poison and dirt in your system.

# CHAPTER 25

# Sunflower Seeds and Grazing

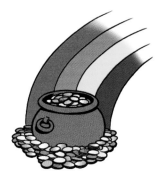

LET ME EMPHASIZE that the Gold Coins are essential to the feeling of fullness that is the basis of my program. This emphasis on fullness began when a number of dieticians started to use the word grazing. This began to alter the mindset of the reader. The old eating-hunger cycle was being replaced by a more level pattern of ingesting five or six meals a day instead of the classic three meals. Studies have shown the very bad effects of the spikes and lows of insulin in the blood which resulted from the large meal followed by hours of fasting. This pattern of hunger was often alleviated by a Coke or candy bar which further exacerbated the spiking.

In my personal life I remember an incident which may have been a factor in leading me to the Fullness Program. A great-uncle of mine was an inveterate smoker. He was told by his doctors that he had incipient emphysema and was in grave danger of lung cancer. He told me how hard it was to try to quit the habit of a lifetime. Nicotine addiction is worse than addiction to hard drugs. These were the days before there were nicotine patches and other aids to break this vicious habit.

My poor great-uncle used to complain to me about the agony of trying to withdraw from nicotine addiction. He told me that he had been smoking for more than sixty years. He recounted other stories that seem incredible in the light of what we know now about smoking. When he was a youngster and visited the doctor for a physical examination the doctor would, of course, offer him a cigarette so they could smoke while they discussed his physical condition. A hostess at a dinner party offered the proper amenities. Along with food and drink she had silver or china containers for cigarettes and matches at each end of each table. Movies showing the good life featured the leading couples smoking through each scene of the development of their relationship.

With this crushing background of nicotine addiction that afflicted our society my uncle found it almost impossible to break the habit. Statistics started to emerge that smoking caused more deaths each year than automobile accidents and heart disease combined. The statistics were alarming, but the chains of this poisonous habit seemed unbreakable. It was then that my great-uncle stumbled upon sunflower seeds.

Uncle Charlie fancied himself a historian. He focused on the Hapsburgs and on Pre-World War I Europe. The most menacing development of that period was the rise of Russian Communism which also spread to China. One of the trivial anecdotes of the period was that the Russian Revolution was fueled by sunflower seeds. The young Communists were fanatic in their hatred of the Tsar. They had little money and had to spend long hours working their underground printing presses to publish their propaganda. The cheapest, most plentiful food available was sunflower seeds. They ate them constantly with three results. First, they felt few hunger pangs because they were eating all day long. Second, they felt a physical well-being which they attributed to the joy of their idealistic work. It may be, however, that their well-being was a result of their continuous eating of this nourishing food. They gorged less at meal-times and became slimmer and trimmer as they lost the excess weight. Finally, most important to my uncle, was the fact that they had less craving for cigarettes which were comparatively expensive. In hindsight we can see that the process of handling the sunflower seed, cracking the shell with one's teeth, extracting the seed with one's tongue, and disposing of the shell, all paralleled the tension-releasing oral activity of cigarette smoking.

This bit of history trivia had two results significant to me. The first is that my great-uncle was able to kick the nicotine habit by substituting a harmless habit. He began by substituting a dozen seeds for every seventh cigarette then for every sixth, and so on. The result for him was that he lost weight and looked great. He also kicked the nicotine addiction by this substitution. He never developed severe emphysema or lung cancer.

The second result of this vignette was that I found it to be a dramatic example of the power of grazing. These young fanatics ate these seeds simply because they were the cheapest food around. The results, however, in regard to their health and weight were impressive. An avid sunflower eater can crack the shells and eat the meat of only three to four ounces of these seeds per day. The steady blood sugar level due to constant eating reduced gorging to a minimum. I must credit these young fanatics of a century ago with giving me an acute insight into the nutritive value of grazing. The continuous eating prevented spiking of the insulin level. Probably of equal import is the continual emotional involvement with food. I attribute a major part of the globesity besetting modern man with his removal from the nutritive process. Historically the human spent a chunk of each day in the elaborate process of obtaining and of preparing each meal. Societies that have maintained this preoccupation with food are not so afflicted with the ravages of globesity. The French are noted for their preoccupation with every aspect of nutrition. Their sauces are egg yolks plus heavy sweet cream. Because of their preoccupation with food they eat far fewer calories than we do and suffer far less high blood pressure, heart disease and obesity than we do. The young Communist fanatics ate these tiny seeds all day simply because they were so cheap. The result however was that they were absorbed with food all day. This gave them a steady insulin level and resulted in health comparable to that of the modern Frenchman. My uncle's nicotine addiction and his stories of the Russian fanatics all contributed to my thinking about the need for a steady insulin level and so contributed to the creation of my Fullness Program.

# CHAPTER 26

# Restaurant Eating

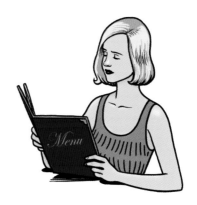

THE NEW WONDER FOODS solve the home menu and the guest menu. These foods don't help with the problem of eating out.

The movie "Super Size Me" showed the horror of some fast foods. Oddly enough it is these "fast food restaurants" that offer the most help to the dieter. Almost all of them offer the basic building blocks of your Festive meal. They offer fat-free dressings for your salads and or vegetables. The fat-free dressing tastes identical to its fatty sister but is a quarter or a fifth as caloric (35 cal as compared to 160 cal). Right there you have a third or a quarter of your dinner calories either salvaged or wasted depending on which dressing you choose.

I don't bother carrying my personal dressings into fast food restaurants because they usually offer the fat-free. Upscale restaurants are not as sophisticated. Since the fat-free is not available I choose their oil and vinegar or better still just plain wine vinegar as a dressing. I've explained in an earlier chapter about the unique position of salad dressing. It is the only food item that can be carried with dignity into the most upscale restaurant. Management knows that many have personal dressings and they also know that using your own dressing will not detract from the price of the meal. They have no question about your carrying your bottle of no-calorie dressing to your table. The caloric savings are impressive.

It would be a mistake to gloss over the no-cal salad dressing lightly. It is obviously a godsend for your salad. The richest salad has few calories. The killer is always the dressing. The mental struggle is whether to eat lettuce and spinach with minimal dressing and so save calories or whether to enjoy the salad with tons of dressing with lots of calories. No-cal or low-cal salad dressing solves the problem for you. It provides great taste with minimal calories. An additional dynamite aspect of this dressing is its use on vegetables. Here we have the parallel problem. Shall I have my vegetables steamed, low calorie and of blah taste? Should I have my vegetable deliciously dripping in butter and other high calorie sauce? Here again the Gordian knot is severed by low-cal or no-cal dressing. You brought this dressing in to dinner with full knowledge and approval of the management. Since it's there already it takes no effort to pour this "salad dressing" onto your vegetables. Now I want to shock you. There have been times that I have extended my victory by having my fish broiled without butter. I used my no cal salad dressing to spice up even the entrée.

My introduction to this section on eating out is also my ending. Upscale restaurants are happy to have you bring in your own salad dressing. They are happy to let you use it on your vegetable and even your entrée. That is just about as far as they will go toward my standard of healthy eating.

I eat at upscale restaurants. I am a member of the prestigious dinner club of New York. I am on a first name basis with many chefs and Maitre D's. Nonetheless I've made no dent on the upscale restaurants in the area of healthy eating. Despite my efforts and those of my friends, they will not compromise on serving only 100 calorie butter instead of the 35 or the 5, 100 calorie mayonnaise instead of the 10, 80 calorie bread instead of the 40, 90 calorie cream cheese instead of the 15. The cream in the coffee is always 70 calories instead of 5. Desserts are always sugar- and fat-filled instead of sugar free. My bottom line about eating out in upscale restaurants is, during your slimming down period in my Fullness Program, "DON'T." After the slimming down period, you will have enough extra calories to be able to eat in these restaurants, if you do so judiciously.

Judicious eating out requires initiative on your part. Tell the waiter to instruct the chef that your fish be broiled without butter and that your salad dressing be served on the side. Choose your vegetables from among the low calorie list that I mention in the supermarket tour. Focus on string beans, broccoli, asparagus and spinach (steamed, of course). Avoid the starchy vegetables like corn, peas and carrots.

Take advantage of the few imaginative creations afforded you in the restaurants. Dunkin Donuts offers an egg white flat bread sandwich at 300 calories and Subway offers a six inch sub that is bread and meat and around 300 calories. As other restauranteurs also join the 21st century take advantage of the high fiber, low calorie dishes they will soon *have* to be offering.

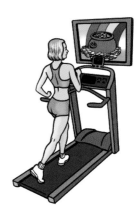

# CHAPTER 27

# Exercise is a Life Sentence

IN MY GRANDFATHER'S DAY there was debate about the advisability of exercise. The historian Engels wrote a famous thesis about the equation of wealth and idleness. His argument was that fashion was designed to prove that the wearer was wealthy and need not work. A lady had white skin to show that she was never in the field. Her wasp waist and high heels and voluminous skirts were additional proof that she could barely move. Engels' most extreme example was the Chinese girl whose feet were bound so tightly at infancy that the bones were deformed and she needed ladies in waiting to help her hobble about throughout her life. I have pictures of some of these poor creatures who were still around until the end of the last century. Even more gross were her husband's fingernails. The aristocratic Mandarin's fingernails were eight inches long or longer. He was helpless. Even his most intimate functions had to be carried out for him by servants.

This heritage of equating aristocracy with immobility died hard. In my grandfather's day there was still debate about the advisability of exercise. That kind of thinking is now of the past. In the last fifteen years, study after study has proved that exercise has many beneficial effects on the heart, muscle tone, etc. There is no doubt that part of a good health regimen is exercise. But, what kind of exercise should you undertake?

The guiding principle of my exercise program must be the same as the guiding principle of my fullness program. It is evident that no diet based on food denial has ever worked. Similarly, no exercise regimen based on sporadic effort and pain can long endure. Remember, exercise is a life sentence.

It has been shown that it is better to be fat than to indulge in the yo-yo ups and downs of dieting and regaining, dieting and regaining. Each yo-yo up and down makes it harder to reach a good set point. There can also be damage to muscle tissue and the bodily organs. The yo-yo effect must be avoided, so the program you undertake must be a lifetime commitment. That is why I object so strongly to the other diets. They may succeed for a while, but what normal person could spend a lifetime on Atkins and Pritikin etc.?

This same philosophy applies to exercise. There are some "jocks" who will exercise hours a day all the days of their lives. Most humans are built of different stuff. They undertake exercise as a result of sporadic resolve. They stick to the program for awhile and then they drop it. Think of the fads of even the last few years. Remember the bowling mania and the indoor tennis mania and the bicycles, and the racquetball, and the roller-skating and the aerobics and the jogging? The new mania is brisk walking. I hope it will last.

Whole industries have been built around these fads. I have been on the inside of them, so I can tell you their formulas. Most of the exercise centers work on the same principle as the dance studios. They advertise heavily and rely on many new enrollments. They know that the majority of their customers follow a standard bell-curve. They come faithfully each day the first week, less by the third week, and drop out after a period of time. They know that only a small percent will use their membership for the full period. They count on the dropout percentage whose spaces will be filled by selling more and more new memberships.

The dropout effect is just as destructive in exercise as the yo-yo up and down is in diet. This is evident in the college athletic stars who worked out strenuously each day when they were at school. The majority could not keep up the pattern of exercise, so the muscle turns to fat. It is sad to see some of these formerly muscular athletes turn into beefy beer drinkers.

The yo-yo effect in exercise is also evident in the vacationer who spends two weeks getting burned by the sun and playing frantically hard after a year of sedentary routine. These poor creatures need a vacation after their vacation. Some of the less fortunate suffer aches, bruises and even heart attacks. It is better to be sedentary all year long than to intersperse your routine of idleness with a short frenzy of athletics.

The solution to the challenge of exercise is inherent in the wording of the challenge. As you define exercise as a life-routine, rather than as a yo-yo up and down, you reject the ordinary exercises forthwith. Who can picture jogging decade after decade? A short period of bad weather can break up the pattern; an illness does the same thing. It is sad to read the statistics about the fallout percentage of exercises in all the various forms of aerobics, calisthenics, jazz dancing, etc. Most drop out of their programs after a period of time. Rarely does one look on exercise as a life sentence.

The answer to finding lifelong exercise is threefold. First, find an exercise that is easy, pleasant, and fun. Anything painful has to be of limited duration and leads to the yo-yo syndrome. Just as the body rejects starvation, the human spirit rejects pain. The painful exertion of many exercises is purposeless. You strive each day to slow down the aging process. You are like the gambler who prays, "Please, God, let me break even today; I need the money."

Expending energy with no reward is painful. Hitler destroyed the spirit of his political prisoners by putting them to useless work. They would dig a pit in the morning and fill the pit up in the afternoon. In short order, most had breakdowns or were suicides.

The serious runners who reach that point that the endorphins give them a "charge" can argue that running is a pleasurable experience. Still, the pain of running is so great that the dropout rate in this discipline is equal to that of the less strenuous forms of exercise.

The first answer to exercise, then, is to break the sense of purposelessness. Stop fighting to make time lessen its ravages on your body. Stop jumping up and down as an end in itself. Find natural patterns where you feel the sense of achievement. Quite simply, walk to the grocery store, if it is a short distance away. Stop paying someone to polish your car; do it yourself.

I see bored friends sitting unhappily while the maids polish the floor and clean the walls. These gals are actually jealous of these servants who are getting their exercise while feeling the reward of accomplishment, while the poor mistress has to get her exercise futily jumping up and down in a boring, expensive aerobics class.

The natural movements of walking, polishing, cleaning, climbing stairs, etc. are by far the best for body tone. I try to do as much physical exertion as I can in the course of a day. I walk at least three miles a day. By now, I never think of mechanical transportation in the city except for very long travel or emergencies. I welcome the chance to walk two or three flights of stairs rather than to take the elevator. I work at housecleaning whenever I can.

This, then, is the first answer. Review your activities of the day. You will find that you can walk a distance instead of riding. You will find that there is work that you can do which you are now delegating to others. You will find at least an hour or two of physical exertion which is pleasurable and purposeful and which you can do for the rest of your life.

The second principle of lifelong exercise is similar to the first. It involves using boring time periods for isometrics. Isometrics, the pressure of muscle against muscle within your body, produces effective, visible results. Simply tensing, and then relaxing, your arm muscles will result in arm muscles that are stronger and more toned.

Isometrics are unique because they can be done invisibly, without equipment, and they help to while away boring time. I have to spend several hours a week in a car. I think and listen to the radio. I also have a pattern of tensing various sets of bodily muscles in a sequence that I have developed over the years. First I tense and relax my shoulder and upper arm muscles 25 times. Then I go down to the stomach and thigh muscles. After 300 tensions and relaxations I have had a workout. I have firmed up my muscles during a time period that would have been waste and boredom. Isometrics serve their valuable function while waiting, or standing in line, or sitting in a subway. They while away the time that would otherwise have been wasted. Best of all you can easily see yourself doing these isometrics for the rest of your life.

The third principle is another lifelong exercise — what I call the television exercycle. The treadmill or exercise bicycle is, in itself, an ideal tool. Twenty minutes on the bicycle increases your heart rate and gets your breathing going with no bad side effects. There is no thumping of the various foot bones (your feet are composed of an amazing number of little bones — more bones than all the rest of your body put together). Your delicate sensitive knees are not subject to strain. You needn't set the bicycle to any real stress. Pick a relaxed setting. The mere pumping of your legs at a decent speed will give you the cardiovascular benefits you need. You can also get a bike with handles that move, so that you can exercise the arm and chest muscles simultaneously. I have this sort of exercycle, and I like it.

Yes, riding the bike itself is an excellent exercise. In itself, though, it has the defect of being purposeless and boring, and therefore painful. The bike would eventually be relegated to the closet with the tennis racquets, rollerskates, etc. No painful exercise is a lifelong exercise. The marvelous thing about the bike though, is that it is completely compatible with television. This changes the painful, transient exercise into a pleasant, lifelong exercise. The bike can easily be set up near a TV set. Watching the 7:00 AM, 6:00 PM or the 11:00 PM news program is a national pastime. It is my daily habit and can easily be projected as a lifelong pattern. Watching television is the magic that transforms exercise from pain to pleasure.

There are variations on this theme. I sometimes read while doing my twenty minutes stint. I have friends who are music buffs and listen to their favorite tunes. I know others who have exercise mechanisms that simulate cross-country skiing or rowing. All of these can work as lifelong exercise patterns if you add the ingredients of television, music or reading.

The essence of my program is that anything that endures must be enjoyable. The painful diets and exercises simply cannot hold you; they lead to the awful yo-yo syndromes in both diet and exercise. The natural, pleasant, harmonious food and exercise programs that I have developed are tied in to your natural desires and patterns. Therefore, they are effective and can be lifelong activities. Enjoy!

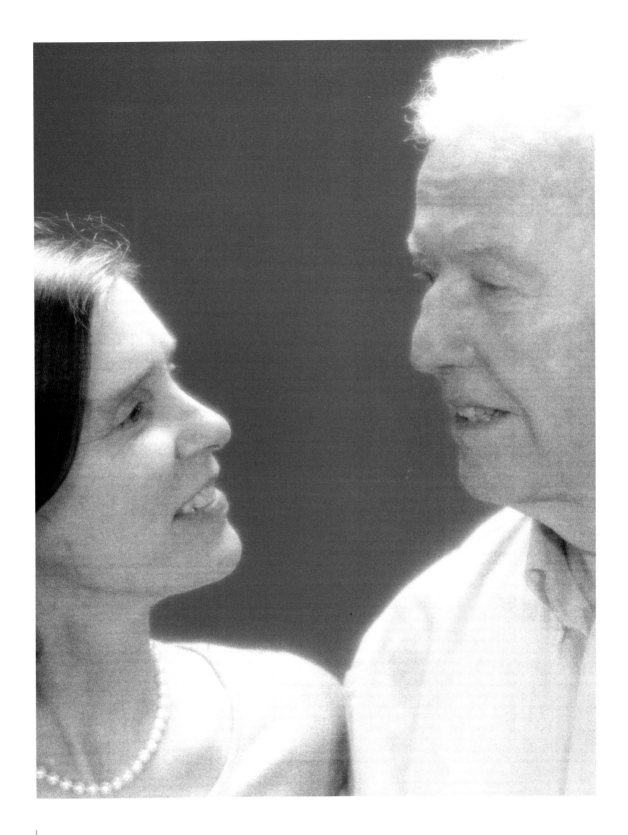

# All Profits Go to Charity

**All profits will be allocated as follows:**

Five percent of the profit from our patent will go to Cornell University in gratitude for its unstinting help in developing it.

The profits from the book we allocate to the F. Cecil Grace Foundation, "Operation: Positive Role Model." We decided that instead of having children of our own, we would try to change the lives of many children for the better. To do this, we established the foundation, which has already awarded more than $250,000 to students at local schools in Westchester and Putnam Counties in New York. Its purpose is to glamorize the good by focusing student dialogue on good rather than on evil. The foundation asks the students to nominate the Good Samaritans who have performed random acts of kindness in the past year. Volunteer student judges then decide on the number of students most worthy. Each student that the judges select receives a $1,000 award.

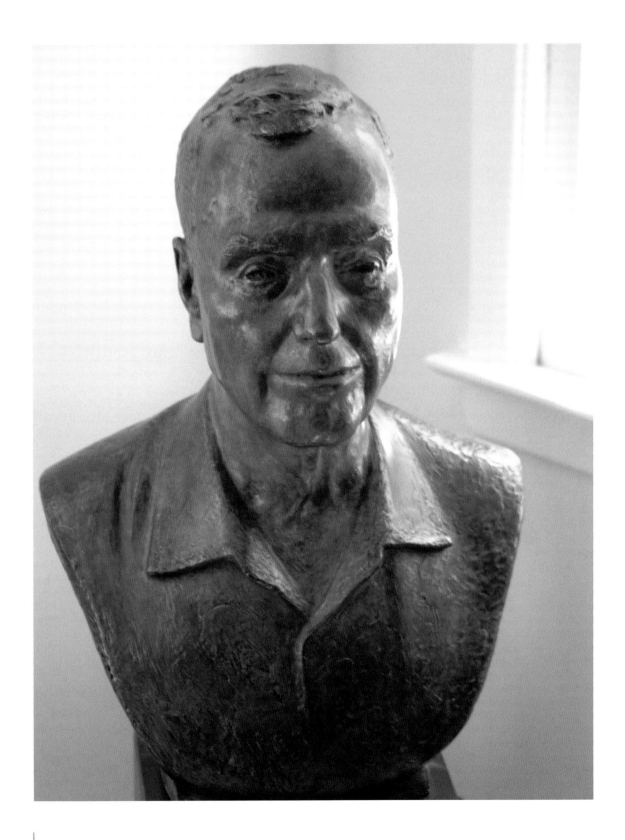

# A Tribute to Our Benefactor

F. Cecil Grace graduated from Harvard as an Electronic Engineer. It was before the Second World War and our country feared enemy invasion. We had no Radar. Cecil was one of the select Electronic Engineers our army chose to study British Radar developments in England and to bring the technical information back to us. He flew and studied Radar in England as part of the ETG (Electronic Training Group).

After the war, Cecil worked with DuMont Television and received a government patent as part of his interest in mechanical music. He has been acutely aware of the major issues of our times. With scholarly levels declining in our schools and with drugs and delinquency burgeoning, Cecil and Boo decided to try to influence the dialogue of our teenagers in the direction of good instead of evil. They founded the F. Cecil Grace "Operation: Positive Role Model" in 2000. Volunteer student judges examine student nominations of other students who have been Good Samaritans over the year. Those students selected by their fellow students each receive a one thousand dollar award. The Positive Role Model Program (PRM) expended over $250,000 in the last six years and is growing rapidly. It is now formally recognized as a not-for-profit Foundation.

The other major problem that Cecil confronted was global obesity which the United Nations pronounced as the single greatest threat to the health of humankind. He sponsored and financed the invention of the Fullness Program and the diet shake and bar. This project received a US patent in 2002.

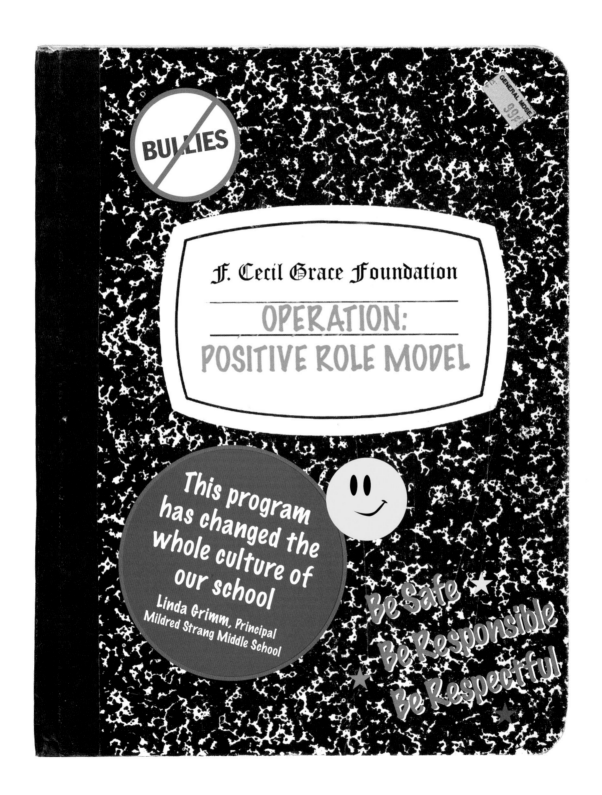

BULLIES

F. Cecil Grace Foundation

OPERATION:
POSITIVE ROLE MODEL

This program has changed the whole culture of our school

Linda Grimm, Principal
Mildred Strang Middle School

Be Safe ★
Be Responsible ★
Be Respectful ★

# Special thanks to:

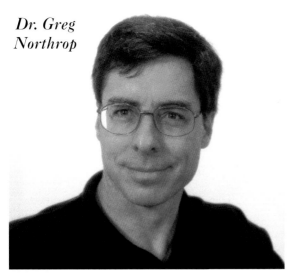

*Dr. Greg Northrop*

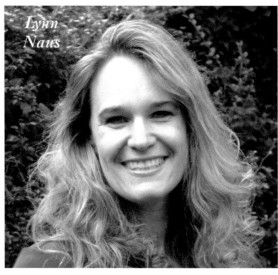

*Lynn Naus*

Linda Grimm
Veronica Hildinger
Theresa Murdock
Lynne Barry
Jenny Monahan
Jeff Nebel
Dr. D'Neapolitano
Dr. Gordon Bruno
Sylvia Epstein
Judge Mark Oxman and family
Clcl Bryant
Bob and Dinah Carroll
Robin Nadell
Tom O'Keefe

Steven Elkman and family
Andres Valdespino
Jeffry Braun
Russell Braun
Herb Cooley
Dr. Andy Rao
Dr. Olga Padilla-Zakour
Stacey Epstein
Emily Wein
Amanda Gilpin
The Research Staff
Mila Bouzinova
Georgianna Vaughan
Frank Silkowski

# Bibliography

Richardson, Vivian. "100 Percent Childhood Obesity Predicted by 2044." Ivanhoe Newswire (2005). 14 June 2007 <http://www.ivanhoe.com/channels/p_channelstory.cfm?storyid=11414>.

Friedman, J.M. "Obesity in the New Millenium." Nature 404 (2000): 632-634.
"Obesity: a Deadly Global Epidemic." NDRI. 2006. 14 June 2007 <http://www.ndri.com/news/obesity_a_deadly_global_epidemic_-51.html>.

"Professor Paul Zimmet." Apollo Life Sciences (2006). 14 June 2007 <http://www.apollolifesciences.com/DiabetesAdvisor.aspx>.

"Scientific Faqs." GeneOb Inc. (2005). 14 June 2007 <http://www.geneob.com/scientificfaqs.html>.

"The World Health Organization Warns of the Rising Threat of Heart Disease and Stroke as Overweight and Obesity Rapidly Increase." WHO. 2007. 14 June 2007 <http://www.who.int/mediacentre/news/releases/2005/pr44/en/index.html>.

"WHO Facilitates Dialogue on Obesity with European Civil Society Networks." WHO/Europa. 1 Apr. 2006. 14 June 2007 <http://www.euro.who.int/PressRoom/pressnotes/20060221_1?language=German>.

Brundtland, Dr. Gro H. Address. Davos, Switzerland. 29 Jan. 2000. na <http://www.who.int/director-general/speeches/2000/english/20000129_davos.html>.

Brody, Jane E. "For Most Trying to Lose Weight, Dieting Only Makes Things Worse." NY Times 23 Nov.1992. <http://query.nytimes.com/gst/fullpage.html?sec=health&res=9E0CE3DB1338F930A15752C1A964958260>.

Garner D M, Wooley C S. "Controversies in Management: Dietary Treatments for Obesity are Ineffective." BMJ. 10 Sept. 1994. <http://www.bmj.com/cgi/content/full/309/6955/655>.

Hirsch, Jules. Interview. ScienceWatch. Mar. 1991. <http://www.sciencewatch.com/interviews/jules_hirsch1.htm>.

Cichoke, Anthony J. The Complete Book of Enzyme Therapy. Avery, 1998. <http://books.google.com/books?id=gJy5neC07YsC&dq=%22complete+book+of+enzyme+therapy%22>.

Fraser, Laura. Ten Pounds in Ten Days. Consumer Health Interactive's. Caremark Inc., 2007. <http://healthresources.caremark.com/topic/dietscams>.

Fraser, Laura. Losing It. Is Obesity A Killer Disease? <http://www.radiancemagazine.com/issues/1998/winter_98/losing_it.html>.

Potts, Aaron M. "Why Diets Don't Work." Ghana. <http://www.ghanaweb.com/GhanaHomePage/women/article.php?ArticleID=26&channel=health_fitness>.

"World Hunger Facts 2006." World Hunger. 8 Sept. 2006. <http://www.worldhunger.org/articles/Learn/world%20hunger%20facts%202002.htm>.

"The Obesity Epidemic: Too Much Food for Thought?" Sports Medicine June 2007. <http://bjsm.bmj.com/cgi/reprint/38/3/360.pdf>.

Lappé, Frances M. "World Hunger: 12 Myths" 3rd ed. Vol. 5. Institute for Food and Development Policy Backgrounder, 1998. Why So Much Hunger? <http://www.mindfully.org/Food/Hunger-12-Myths.htm>.

Obesity Around the World." Unilever. 2007. <http://www.unilever.com/ourvalues/nutritionhygien-epersonalcare/nutrition/weight_management/a_global_challenge/>.

"Obesity Pandemic Engulfing World: Experts." AFP 2005. <http://www.breitbart.com/article.php?id=060903083715.f0p6azce&show_article=1>.

Gardner, Gary. "Underfed and Overfed: the Global Epidemic of Malnutrition." Worldwatch Paper. <http://www.worldwatch.org/node/840>.

Swaminathan, M. S. Interview with Andreas Stauffer. SDC. 23 Aug. 2005. <http://72.14.209.104/search?q=cache:uBBPF77dAgAJ:www.sdc.admin.ch/en/Dossiers/Event_Traverse/ressources/resource_en_25169.pdf+Prof.+Swaminathan+let%E2%80%99s+refer+to+the+words+of+Gandhi+to+begin+this&hl=en&ct=clnk&cd=1&gl=us>.

Squires, Nick. "Overweight People Now Outnumber the Hungry." Telegraph 16 Aug. 2006. <http://www.telegraph.co.uk/news/main.jhtml?xml=/news/2006/08/15/wfat15.xml>.

Montanari, Massimo. "Food is Culture." Colombia University Press (2006). <http://www.columbia.edu/cu/cup/publicity/montanariexcerpt.html>.

Calle, Eugenia E., Carmen Rodriguez, Kimberly W. Thurmond, and Michael J. Thun. "Overweight, Obesity, and Mortality From Cancer in a Prospectively Studied Cohort of U.S. Adults." The New England Journal of Medicine 348 (2003). <http://content.nejm.org/cgi/content/abstract/348/17/1625?journalcode=nejm&minscore=5000&qbe=nejm%3BNEJMsb020030&searchid=1083679923754_5493&FIRSTINDEX=0&minscore=5000&journalcode=nejm>.

Finkelstein, Eric. The Economics of Obesity. RTI International. 1-23. 15 June 2007 <www.yaleruddcenter.org/download.aspx?id=79>.

"Economics of Obesity, Getting Kids to Eat Fruit and Veggies Focus of Two New UAB Studies." UAB Media Relations 22 Nov. 2002. <http://main.uab.edu/show.asp?durki=71818>.

"Statistics Related to Overweight and Obesity." Weight-Control Information Network. 2006. <http://win.niddk.nih.gov/statistics/index.htm#what>.

O'neill, Molly. "A Growing Movement Fights Diets Instead of Fat." NY Times 12 Apr. 1992. <http://query.nytimes.com/gst/fullpage.html?sec=health&res=9E0CE0DC133AF931A25757C0A9649 58260&n=Top%2fNews%2fHealth%2fDiseases%2c%20Conditions%2c%20and%20Health%20Topics %2fBulimia>.

Kolata, Gina. "Diet and Lose Weight? Scientists Say 'Prove It!'" NY Times 4 Jan. 2005. <http://www.nytimes.com/2005/01/04/health/nutrition/04fat.html?ex=1262667600&en=572cc222d1097 7e0&ei=5088&partner=rssnyt>.

"Sumo Wrestlers: This is How You Get Fat." Diet Blog (2005). <http://www.diet-blog.com/archives/2005/03/21/sumo_wrestlers_this_is_how_you_get_fat.php>.

"Sumo East and West." Discovery Channel. 2007. <http://www.discoverychannelasia.com/sumo/become_a_sumo_wrestler/index.shtml>.

Nishizawa, T, I Akaoka, Y Nishida, Y Kawaguchi, and E Hayashi. "Some Factors Related to Obesity in the Japanese Sumo Wrestler." The American Journal of Clinical Nutrition 29 (1976). <http://www.ajcn.org/cgi/content/abstract/29/10/1167>.

Lundberg, Da, Ra Nelson, Hw Wahner, and Jd Jones. "Protein Metabolism in the Black Bear Before and During Hibernation." Mayo Clin Proc. (1976): 716-22. <http://www.ncbi.nlm.nih.gov/sites/entrez?cmd=Retrieve&db=PubMed&list_uids=825685&dopt=Ab stract>.

Angier, Natalie. "Built for the Arctic: a Species' Splendid Adaptations." NY Times 27 Jan. 2004. <http://query.nytimes.com/gst/fullpage.html?sec=health&res=9C05E1DF1438F934A15752C0A9629C 8B63>.

FAO Report: Enough Food in the Future—Without Genetically Engineered Crops. FAO. UCSUSA, 2000. <http://www.ucsusa.org/food_and_environment/genetic_engineering/world-food-supply.html>.

Tackett, Chad. "Diets Don't Work!" Free Weight Loss. <http://www.freeweightloss.com/article21.html>.

"Heart Disease, Liver Disease and Other Risks of Obesity." Obesity Focused. <http://www.obesity-focused.com/articles/effects-of-obesity/obesity-and-disease-risks.php>.

"No Need to Diet and Exercise to Lose Weight." Reuters Health 22 Feb. 2002. <http://www.reuters.com/article/healthNews/idUSTON20527420070222>.

"Do You Know the Health Risks of Being Overweight?" Weight-Control Information Network. Nov. 2004. <http://win.niddk.nih.gov/publications/health_risks.htm>.

"'Obesity a World-Wide Hazard'" <u>BBC NEWS</u> 22 Dec. 2002. <http://news.bbc.co.uk/1/hi/health/1082739.stm>.

"AOA Fact Sheets." <u>American Obesity Associatiob</u>. 2002. <http://obesityusa.org/subs/fastfacts/Health_Effects.shtml>.

Hellmich, Nanci. "Obesity Threatens Life Expectancy." <u>USA Today</u> 17 Mar. 2005. <http://www.usatoday.com/educate/health/articles/art2.htm>.

"Study: Obesity an Independent Risk Factor for Fatal Pulmonary Embolism." <u>Obesity Week</u> 4 (2005). <http://www.obesityweek.org/members/Vol4/News/091005.htm>.

Belkin, Lisa. "The School-Lunch Test." <u>NY Times</u> 20 Aug. 2006. <http://www.nytimes.com/2006/08/20/magazine/20lunches.html?ex=1182052800&en=99880740ba80f28b&ei=5070>.

"Facts About Low-Calorie Sweeteners." <u>International Food Information Council</u>. May 2006. <http://ific.org/publications/factsheets/lcsfs.cfm>.
White, Sarah. "ICO 2006: Obesity World'S Biggest Health Problem." <u>Obesity Conferences</u> (2006). <http://calorielab.com/news/categories/obesity-conferences/>.
"Health Topics." Why Diets Don't Work: The Myths that Make us Massive. 1999. <http://www.refityourself.com/refit/healthtopics_article5.html>.

Obesity Becoming Major Global Problem." NewsMax. 10 May 2004. <http://www.newsmax.com/archives/articles/2004/5/9/150423.shtml>.

Schmidhuber, Josef. "The Growing Global Obesity Problem: Some Policy Options to Address It." <u>Journal of Agricultural and Development Economics</u> 1 (2004): 273-275. <http://209.85.165.104/search?q=cache:6_UdiKKSBHQJ:ftp://ftp.fao.org/docrep/fao/007/ae228e/ae228e00.pdf+It+took+more+than+a+century+before+the+agro-industrial+revolution+started+to+reach&hl=en&ct=clnk&cd=2&gl=us>.

"Fighting Hunger Today Could Help Prevent Obesity Tomorrow." FAO Newsroom. 11 Feb. 2004. <http://www.fao.org/newsroom/en/news/2004/36847/index.html>.

McGovern, George. "The Real Cost of Hunger." <u>UN Chronicle</u> 3 (2001). <http://www.un.org/Pubs/chronicle/2001/issue3/0103p24.html>.

"Food Rights." Actionaid. 2006. <http://www.actionaid.org/main.aspx?PageID=24>.

UCLA. "Dieting Does Not Work, Researchers Report." Science Daily. 5 Apr. 2007. <http://www.sciencedaily.com/releases/2007/04/070404162428.htm>.

"Where Diets Go Wrong!" Health Recipes. <http://www.healthrecipes.com/consumer_diets.htm>.

"Learn About the Top 5 Diet Scams." KPHO Phoenix. 2006. <http://www.kpho.com/health/10469338/detail.html>.

"Report: Scientists Still Seeking Cure for Obesity." the Onion. 14 July 2004.
<http://www.theonion.com/content/node/30630>.

Kutty, Suhil. "That in a Nutshell is the Obese World We Live in, and Which Future Corpulent Generations." Khaleej Times 22 June 2004.
<http://www.khaleejtimes.com/DisplayArticleNew.asp?section=citytimes&xfile=data/citytimes/2004/june/citytimes_june139.xml>.

"Up to 70% of Gulf Women are Obese." Middle East Online. 29 Sept. 2005. <http://www.middle-east-online.com/english/Default.pl?id=14663>.

Zelman, Kathleen. "Global Gaining Leading to 'Globesity' Crisis." FOXNews. 26 Oct. 2005.
<http://www.foxnews.com/story/0,2933,173456,00.html>.

MacRae, Fiona. "Diets Damage Health, Shows Biggest Ever Study." Daily Mail. 10 Apr. 2007.
<http://www.dailymail.co.uk/pages/live/articles/news/news.html?in_article_id=447651&in_page_id=1770&ct=5>.

"Why Diets Don't Work." Southern Connecticut State University. <http://www.southernct.edu/womenscenter/whydietsdontwork/>.

"Diet Damage." The State News. 17 Jan. 2006.
<http://www.statenews.com/article.phtml?pk=33991>.

"Obesity Seen as Greatest Threat." BBC NEWS. 31 Mar. 2004. <http://news.bbc.co.uk/1/hi/programmes/real_story/3562321.stm>.

"The War on Fat." Men's Fitness. Oct. 2004.
<http://findarticles.com/p/articles/mi_m1608/is_9_20/ai_n6242975>.

"Obesity Epidemic 'Bigger Threat Than Terrorism'" The Guardian. 3 Mar. 2006.
<http://www.guardian.co.uk/usa/story/0,,1722464,00.html>.

Saletan, William. "Please Don't Feed the People." The Washington Post. 3 Sept. 2006.
<http://www.washingtonpost.com/wp-dyn/content/article/2006/09/01/AR2006090101400.html>.

Goodstein, Ellen. "10 Secrets of the Weight-Loss Industry." Bankrate.
<http://www.bankrate.com/brm/news/advice/20040113a1.asp>.

Strom, Stephanie. "$500 Million Pledged to Fight Childhood Obesity." NY Times. 4 Apr. 2007.
<http://www.nytimes.com/2007/04/04/health/04obesity.html?ei=5070&en=46c48b6b5653bec5&ex=1182484800&adxnnl=1&adxnnlx=1182349020-OGhVoG5OS7AkIVXUf1/N1Q>.

Landon, Thomas Jr. "Disney Says It Will Link Marketing to Nutrition." NY Times.
<http://www.nytimes.com/2006/10/17/business/media/17disney.html?ex=1182484800&en=ce09b1a6f9c59bfc&ei=5070>.

Kipnis, Laura. "America's Waistline." <u>Slate</u> 28 Oct. 2005. <http://www.slate.com/id/2128999/>.

Sorkin, Andrew R. "Nestlé to Buy Jenny Craig, Betting Diets are on Rise." NY Times. 19 June 2006. <http://www.nytimes.com/2006/06/19/business/worldbusiness/19deal.html?ex=1308369600&en=639ab cb011624958&ei=5088&partner=rssnyt&emc=rss>.

"EU Alarmed by Spread of Obesity." BBC NEWS. 15 Mar. 2005. <http://news.bbc.co.uk/2/hi/europe/4351509.stm>.

Sofsian, Damien. "What You Need to Know About Obesity." Ezine @rticles. 27 July 2006. <http://ezinearticles.com/?What-You-Need-To-Know-About-Obesity&id=254779&opt=print>.

"Obesity - Our Ticking Time Bomb." Sunderland Echo. 15 Mar. 2007. <http://www.sunderlande-cho.com/ViewArticle.aspx?SectionID=1512&articleid=2123254>.

"FAD DIETS." <u>IVillage</u>. <http://magazines.ivillage.com/goodhousekeeping/diet/plans/arti-cles/0,,284559_290212-1,00.html>.

Streib, Lauren. "World's Fattest Countries." Forbes. 8 Feb. 2007. <http://www.forbes.com/2007/02/07/worlds-fattest-countries-forbeslife-cx_ls_0208worldfat.html>.

Brody, Jane E. <u>Jane Brody's Nutrition Book</u>. New York, Bantam Books, 1981, 1987. pg 297.

*Boo's fullness program is a promising new tool in the fight against obesity. Finally, we have a diet plan that allows you to lose weight and feel* full, *not* hungry.

*Michael S. Wein M.D.*
*Undergraduate – University of Pennsylvania Magna Cum Laude*
*Medical – NYU School of Medicine*
*Residency – Harvard's Beth Israel Deaconess Medical Center*
*Board Certified in Internal Medicine by American Board of Internal Medicine*
*Member of the Amercian College of Physicians*

*As a physician I have seen many people struggle with obesity. Most diets have resulted in only modest success and temporary weight loss. The Graces have introduced a simple concept that makes good physiological sense. The* Slim Satisfied and Sexy *diet keeps the stomach full with good-tasting low calorie alternatives. This is such a simple concept and is one of the ideas that make the diet so appealing.*

*Harvey Gorrin M.D.*

*I was very fortunate to read your draft of* Slim Satisfied and Sexy *and was so very intrigued that I worked in some of your tips… I have lost over 15 pounds and now exercise daily. The weight has come off steadily, and with little deprivation. I found one product after another as each one pleasantly surprised me. How easy it has been to trade in high fat, needless foods and condiments and see little changes result in big losses. I have now been able to lose my "married and happy fat." Your program has transformed how I look at and enjoy food, and the more I lose, the more it motivates me to keep exploring new options. You have been a blessing to me!*

*Victoria, Yorktown Heights, NY*